Memory and Language Impairment in Children and Adults

New Perspectives

Editor

Ronald B. Gillam, PhD
Associate Professor
The University of Texas at Austin
Austin, Texas

Articles selected
Editor:

AN ASPEN PUBLICATION®
Aspen Publishers, Inc.
Gaithersburg, Maryland
1998

Library of Congress Cataloging-in-Publication Data

Memory and language impairment in children and adults: new perspectives/editor, Ronald B. Gillam.
p. cm.
Includes bibliographical references and index.
ISBN 0-8342-1213-7
1. Language disorders. 2. Language disorders in children.
3. Memory. I. Gillam, Ronald B. (Ronald Bradley), 1955– .
RC423.M45 1998
616.85'5—dc21
98-27277
CIP

Orders: (800) 638-8437
Customer Service: (800) 234-1660

About Aspen Publishers • For more than 35 years, Aspen has been a leading professional publisher in a variety of disciplines. Aspen's vast information resources are available in both print and electronic formats. We are committed to providing the highest quality information available in the most appropriate format for our customers. Visit Aspen's Internet site for more information resources, directories, articles, and a searchable version of Aspen's full catalog, including the most recent publications: **http://www.aspenpublishers.com**
Aspen Publishers, Inc. • The hallmark of quality in publishing
Member of the worldwide Wolters Kluwer group.

Editorial Services: Denise H. Coursey
Library of Congress Catalog Card Number: 98-27277
ISBN: 0-8342-1213-7

Printed in the United States of America

1 2 3 4 5

To my parents, Ron and Jean Gillam

Table of Contents

Contributors

Tamiko Azuma, PhD
Department of Psychology
Arizona State University
Tempe, AZ

Kathryn A. Bayles, PhD
Professor
Department of Speech and Hearing
    Sciences
Institute for Neurogenic
    Communication Disorders
University of Arizona
Tuscon, AZ

Nelson Cowan, PhD
Middlebush Professor
Department of Psychology
University of Missouri
Columbia, MO

Susan Ellis Weismer, PhD
Department of Communicative
    Disorders and Waisman Center
University of Wisconsin
Madison, WI

Barbara B. Fazio, PhD
Assistant Professor
Speech and Hearing Sciences
Indiana University
Bloomington, IN

Ronald B. Gillam, PhD
Associate Professor
Department of Communication
    Sciences and Disorders
The University of Texas at Austin
Austin, TX

Douglas Herrmann, PhD
Professor and Chairperson
Psychology Department
Indiana State University
Terre Haute, IN

Judith A. Hudson, PhD
Department of Psychology
Rutgers, The State University of
    New Jersey
New Brunswick, NJ

Judith Hutchinson, PhD
St. David's Rehabilitation Center
Austin, TX

Thomas P. Marquardt, PhD
Department of Communication
    Sciences and Disorders
The University of Texas at Austin
Austin, TX

**James W. Montgomery, PhD,
    CCC-SLP**
Assistant Professor
Division of Speech and Hearing
    Sciences
University of North Carolina at
    Chapel Hill
Chapel Hill, NC

Rita C. Naremore, PhD
Professor
Speech and Hearing Sciences
Indiana University
Bloomington, IN

Rick Parenté, PhD
Professor of Psychology
Towson State University
Towson, MD
Adjunct Associate Professor of
    Physiology
University of Maryland—Dental
    School
Baltimore, MD

Anne van Kleeck, PhD
Professor
Department of Communication
    Sciences and Disorders
The University of Texas at Austin
Austin, TX

**M. Lorraine Wynn-Dancy, MS,
    MA, CCC-SLP**
Department of Communication
    Sciences and Disorders
The University of Texas at Austin
Austin, TX

Preface

This book contains the contributions to two issues of *Topics in Language Disorders,* Volume 17:1, entitled "Working Memory and Language Impairment: New Perspectives," and Volume 18:1, entitled "Long-Term Memory and Language Impairment: Evaluation and Treatment Issues."

I would like to thank the authors of the articles that are reprinted here. I invited them to contribute to the *TLD* issues on memory because they are highly respected experts who have unique perspectives on relationships among memory, language, and language disorders and the implications these perspectives have for assessment and intervention of children and adults with language impairments.

I am grateful to a number of dedicated professionals at Aspen Publishers, Inc. Katharine Butler, the editor of *Topics in Language Disorders* offered a great deal of advice, encouragement, and assistance during the 2 years that we worked together on the *TLD* issues. I offer my special thanks to Amy Martin, who originally suggested this project, and to Denise Coursey, who shepherded it to press.

My own work on this project was made possible by a Clinical Investigator Development Award from the National Institute on Deafness and Other Communication Disorders. My wife and children (Lauri, Sara, and Jenn) continually grant me a great deal of time to pursue this and many other academic projects. They contribute in other ways as well. It is my good fortune to be married to an excellent editor. In addition, Sara and Jennifer discuss comprehension, memory, and academics with me regularly, attempt various study strategies that I suggest, and provide their perspectives on my assessment and intervention ideas. I am extremely indebted to my family for their understanding, their patience, and their sage advice.

Introduction

During the seven years that I worked as a speech-language pathologist in the public schools, I became increasingly interested in the academic difficulties experienced by children with language impairments. These children frequently showed learning deficits that seemed to occur at the intersection of language and memory. For example, a teacher once remarked to me, "It seems like it takes Curt twice as long as everyone else to learn something, and half as long as anyone else to forget it."

Difficulties with storing, retaining, recalling, and reporting information place individuals with language impairments at a significant disadvantage in academic, vocational, and social situations. Language assessment and intervention strategies that take into account how cognitive systems such as memory contribute to learning and using language should provide a useful foundation for improving the communication abilities of children and adults with language impairments.

Recently, researchers have made real progress in understanding various memory systems and how they influence language development and academic achievement. This book focuses on recent developments in the understanding of short-term memory, working memory, and long-term memory, and their relationship to language comprehension, lexical development, early academic development, later academic development, and communication following brain damage. Each chapter applies theoretical and research advances in memory to assessment and intervention issues that are important to clinicians who treat children and adults with language impairments.

Working memory, the topic of the first section of the book, often refers to a set of attention, storage, planning, and mental representation processes that "work" together during mental activities such as problem solving and reasoning. Working memory involves immediate recall (short-term memory), but it also involves aspects of long-term memory that are activated at a given moment. Perhaps the most famous model of working memory is Baddeley's phonological loop model (Baddeley, 1986). According to this model, sounds are first represented as sets of sensory features known as *memory traces*. The trace contains information about the order of sounds and their relationship to one another. This lingering trace facilitates recall by providing more time to construct a phonetic code of the sounds. These ordered representations can be compared with what is already known (activated parts of long-term memory), and they can be reactivated during rehearsal and recall processes. The capacity of working memory (the amount of information that can be processed at any given time) is limited by the speed with which information is activated, the specificity of mental representations, the ability to focus and sustain mental energy, and the ability to report experiences effortlessly.

There are alternatives to Baddeley's model of working memory, most notably a model by Nelson Cowan (Cowan, 1984, 1988, 1993, 1995; Cowan, Cartwright, Winterowd, & Sherk, 1987) that includes relationships among attention, sensory storage, short-term storage, central executive functions, and long-term storage. In Chapter 1, Nelson Cowan summarizes recent empirical and theoretical advances in the understanding of short-term and working memory, and provides information about some clinical applications suggested by this research. The remainder of the chapters in the first section concern limitations in working memory and the ways that memory limitations affect various aspects of language in children and adults with language impairments. In Chapter 2, Jim Montgomery describes his recent research on working memory and language comprehension. Susan Ellis Weismer explains how capacity limitations in memory affect lexical development in Chapter 3. Next, in Chapter 4, Barbara Fazio discusses rote memory and its effect on counting and rhyming development. In Chapter 5, Anne van Kleeck and I describe one approach to dealing with relationships between working memory and phonological awareness. Finally, Rick Parenté and Douglas Herrmann provide practical suggestions for teaching memory strategies during cognitive rehabilitation in Chapter 6.

Working memory is not the only memory system that relates to communication. Long-term memory, which consists of processes involved in recalling information for days, months, or years at a time, influences communicative functions such as sharing prior experiences with others, telling stories, and explaining the steps involved in completing activities. Unlike working memory, long-term memory has a very large capacity, requires specific mental attention during storage and recall, and is not very susceptible to outside interference.

Studies of animals, unimpaired human subjects, and individuals with various cognitive and communication disorders support the idea that there are different kinds of long-term memory systems. These memory systems differ according to the cognitive processes involved in remembering or forgetting, the kind of information processed, and the neural mechanisms used in processing.

Long-term memory is most often divided into declarative or nondeclarative systems. According to Schacter and Tulving (1994), there are two declarative memory systems (semantic memory and episodic memory) and one nondeclarative memory system (procedural memory). *Semantic memory* concerns knowledge and beliefs about facts and concepts. However, semantic memory doesn't apply only to words. Activities like recognizing faces and recalling something about the people we know also make use of the semantic memory system. *Episodic memory* (also referred to as *event* or *autobiographical memory*) is used for recording and recollecting experiences. The episodic memory system certainly involves semantic memory, but it goes beyond the boundaries of semantic memory because it involves associations between causal and temporal aspects of experiences. *Procedural memory* (also known as *nondeclarative memory*) is less well specified. Despite what its name might suggest, this type of memory does not concern the ability to recall the steps that are involved in a process. Rather, procedural memory relates to automatic recall of motor and cognitive skills such as putting together a jigsaw puzzle or completing a maze.

The second section of the book concerns various aspects of long-term memory as they relate to language disorders. In Chapter 7, Judith Hudson and I discuss factors that have been shown to facilitate children's event memories. We provide evidence that language and memory interact dynamically within and across encoding, storage, retrieval, and reporting processes. We also suggest assessment and intervention procedures that are consistent with our dynamic perspective.

Event memory plays an important role in narration. In Chapter 8, Rita Naremore explains how long-term memories of events are mentally represented as scripts that provide the underlying frameworks for personal and fictional stories. She provides a number of case vignettes that demonstrate ways to determine where breakdowns in narration might occur.

Long-term memory plays a critical role in learning. In Chapter 9, Lorraine Wynn-Dancy and I describe two metacognitive strategies that we have taught to adolescents to facilitate memory and comprehension of expository texts and other academic materials. We believe adolescents need to act strategically if they are to be successful in a variety of learning contexts, and we present a method for facilitating the development of strategic problem solving.

The last two chapters in this section concern long-term memory in patients with acquired language disorders. In Chapter 10, Judith Hutchinson and Thomas Marquardt describe how to differentiate among sources of cognitive impairment. They also explain the implications of their assessment approach for treating memory disorders that result from traumatic brain injury. In Chapter 11, Tamiko Azuma and Kathryn Bayles profile the memory difficulties that are commonly seen in individuals with dementia resulting from Alzheimer's, Parkinson's, and Lewy body disease. They also describe techniques for assessing and treating language and memory impairments in patients with dementia.

Finally, in an epilogue, I discuss the memory requirements in typical language intervention contexts with children and adults. I present a simple model of the dynamic relationships among working memory, long-term memory, information processing systems, language ability, and world knowledge. I also summarize six language intervention principles and activities that were proposed in the first two sections of the book.

The ultimate goal of language intervention is to improve our clients' ability to function in the social, educational, and vocational contexts that are part of their world. When children have difficulty recounting their personal experiences, when adolescents provide simplistic summaries of expository texts, or when adults appear to be confused about the details or the sequence of events, they are evidencing difficulties that lie at the intersection of language and memory. Language specialists who wish to have an impact on functional communication should attend to relationships between language and memory processes in their assessment and intervention practices. The authors of the articles that are reprinted in this book have provided information and informed clinical suggestions that should be useful for such endeavors.

REFERENCES

Baddeley, A.D. (1986). *Working memory*. Oxford, England: Oxford University Press.

Cowan, N. (1984). On short and long auditory stores. *Psychological Bulletin, 96,* 341–370.

Cowan, N. (1988). Evolving conceptions of memory storage, selective attention, and their mutual constraints within the human information-processing system. *Psychological Bulletin, 104*(2), 163–191.

Cowan, N. (1993). Activation, attention, and short-term memory. *Memory and Cognition, 21*(2), 162–167.

Cowan, N. (1995). *Attention and memory: An integrated framework.* New York: Oxford University Press.

Cowan, N., Cartwright, C., Winterowd, C., & Sherk, M. (1987). An adult model of pre-school children's speech memory. *Memory and Cognition, 15*(6), 511–517.

Schacter, D.L., & Tulving, E. (1994). What are the memory systems of 1994? In D.L. Schacter & E. Tulving (Eds.), *Memory systems 1994* (pp. 1–38). Cambridge, MA: MIT Press.

PART I

Working Memory and Language Impairment

1

Short-Term Memory, Working Memory, and Their Importance in Language Processing

Nelson Cowan

Short-term memory and working memory play central roles in language use; indeed, they play central roles in just about every human activity. The basic phenomenon motivating an interest in these types of memory is that—in contrast to the vast wealth of information that one can store for the long term—one can think about or "keep in mind" only a few ideas at a time, a human limitation that was noted near the beginning of experimental psychology (James, 1890) and again near the beginning of modern cognitive psychology (Miller, 1956). The mental faculty that holds this small amount of information was termed *primary memory* by James and *short-term memory* by cognitive psychologists.

Although its capability is so limited, short-term memory is critical for thought. For example, it is impossible to comprehend a word within conversation or text without keeping in mind the necessary background information established by the prior words in the sentence, and often by preceding sentences. Similarly, it is impossible to speak or write a word of discourse without keeping in mind the intent of the sentence, what the listener or reader has been told thus far, and the goal for making the intended meaning clear. Thus, for language reception, short-term memory serves the role of accumulating information while comprehension occurs. For language production, it serves the role of maintaining information while planning happens. For any type of reasoning or problem solving, typically there are premises or assumptions that must be held in mind if successful thinking is to occur.

Top Lang Disord 1996;17(1):1–18

This general use of short-term memory in human thought is what led to the second major concept to be discussed: *working memory*. Baddeley and Hitch (1974) coined this term to refer to the temporary memory used in information processing. It is not as if one has short-term memory in one area of the brain and working memory in another. Instead, short-term memory refers to a vivid form of memory that lasts for only a few seconds after one receives a stimulus or thinks of something, and working memory usually refers to short-term memory when it is used to solve a problem or perform a task.

The tasks that have been taken to define short-term memory are those that have appeared to indicate a difference among the types of information that can be held in the short- versus long-term memory. For example, Sachs (1967) found that the exact phrasing of a sentence usually is forgotten quickly after the sentence is comprehended, whereas the memory of its gist or meaning persists much longer, perhaps indefinitely. This type of finding has led to the notion of verbal short-term memory as rich, detailed, and temporarily held information about the surface properties of language (a view that has been expounded more fully by Baddeley, 1986). When information is needed temporarily in the service of the current mental activity, that information (if successfully retrieved) is said to be held in working memory.

Current knowledge about short-term and working memory can be useful to speech-language clinicians. Children with language impairments often have deficiencies in short-term or working memory that cannot be attributed to the language problem itself. This finding potentially can lead to the improved diagnosis of particular subtypes of language disorders and eventually to improved treatments. However, such new theoretical developments—if applied with too much blind trust—might lead to useless or harmful misapplications as easily as they might lead to effective ones. A deeper understanding of the original research thus is needed to make sound practical applications.

Thus, this chapter summarizes the empirical research basis underlying the concepts of short-term and working memory and explains how these concepts have been applied to language impairments. Then some recent developments in understanding short-term and working memory are examined. Speech-language pathologists are urged to be cautious when interpreting the clinically relevant literature and to analyze it in depth.

THE BASIC FINDINGS WITH PARTICIPANTS WITHOUT LANGUAGE DISORDERS

Short-term memory

One fundamental question is whether the term *short-term memory* should be used to refer to a temporary neural activation of information or to one's current awareness of the information. A second question is what information persists in short-term memory and for how long. These questions will be addressed.

Activation versus awareness

The basic, seemingly straightforward concept of short-term memory has been the focus of considerable debate recently. No one denies that the amount of information that can be held in mind at one time is limited. However, there is a debate about what "held in mind" means. One meaning is that the neural representation of the information—whatever it consists of—is in a particularly active or accessible state at the moment (Hebb, 1949). A second meaning is that the person is consciously aware of the information at the moment (James, 1890). In more extensive recent reviews of short-term memory and other aspects of information processing, Cowan (1988, 1995) claimed that those two meanings of short-term memory cannot be synonymous because there is evidence of the activation of information without the subject's prior awareness of it. To cite one example of activation without awareness, some investigators have found that processing of a target word is speeded up when it is preceded by a semantically related word, or "prime." For example, priming from the word *student* occurs when it is followed by a related word such as *teacher*, which can be named or identified more quickly than it could if a word such as *student* had not been presented first. Balota (1983), Marcel (1983), and others have followed some of the primes closely with visual patterns that rendered subjects unable to perceive whether the prime word was presented at all or to identify it. Nevertheless, these "unconsciously processed" primes had the same effect as consciously processed primes.

To cite a second and different example of activation without awareness, Wood and Cowan (1995) refined and replicated a classic experiment by Moray (1959). In these experiments, words presented to one ear were to be ignored while the subject repeated, or "shadowed," a passage presented to the other ear. The occurrence of the subject's name in the ignored channel often resulted in later recall of the name. Wood and Cowan also found that some subjects hesitated or made errors in shadowing shortly after their name was presented, but not after another person's name was presented. Only those who stumbled in shadowing proceeded to recall the name. It appears that when some subjects heard their own name, its memory representation was automatically activated, recruiting the subject's attention away from the shadowing task temporarily.

There is still controversy concerning whether information can be activated without any involvement of conscious awareness (for an argument against this, see Holender, 1986; but for recent evidence in favor of it, see Bentin, Kutas, & Hillyard, 1995). However, the evidence seems sufficient to establish the point that activation and awareness are separate mechanisms (Cowan, 1988, 1995). The notion is that there is a small portion of the information in long-term memory that is in a current state of heightened activation and that only a subset of that active information is currently in conscious awareness. For an example of this arrangement of mental faculties, imagine that you are trying to remember a phone number. It does not seem that you could be consciously aware of all seven numbers at one time, but the fact that all of the items are easily accessible for a short time suggests that they all are active in memory at one time.

Persistence of information in short-term memory

The activation or the awareness of information does not last long unless the subject works hard to keep it in mind (e.g., through verbal rehearsal). One of the first studies to verify this point was that of Peterson and Peterson (1959). On each trial they presented three consonants followed by a period of up to 18 seconds, during which subjects engaged in a distracting task and counted backward by threes to prevent them from silently rehearsing the three consonants. The learning theories of the time predicted that three consonants followed only by such dissimilar material should be recalled easily. However, memory for the consonants declined rapidly across test delays. The items were said to be held in a short-term storage faculty that permitted only a limited persistence. The consonants themselves also clearly were in long-term memory as general knowledge, but the episodic record of the trial (the fact that those particular consonants were presented on a particular trial) presumably could be retrieved only from a short-term memory store that could remain only if the test delay was short enough.

Glanzer and Cunitz (1966) distinguished between short- and long-term memory on the basis of a task in which every list of words presented was to be recalled immediately in any order. This method produces much better recall of the first and last few items in the list compared with the medial items. These advantages are known as the *primacy* and *recency effects,* respectively. However, when an 18-second-long distracting task was placed between the list and the recall period—so that recall was no longer immediate—the primacy effect remained intact but the recency effect disappeared. The authors' explanation was that the primacy and recency effects come from different mechanisms. The primacy effect supposedly is caused by efficient covert rehearsal, which becomes increasingly difficult to perform on a cumulative basis as the number of items to rehearse increases. In contrast, the recency effect is a result of the last few items being held in a short-term storage faculty that cannot survive a long, distractor-filled delay.

The findings discussed in this section converge on the notion that short-term memory lasts about 20 to 30 seconds. However, it is possible that the estimate has been extended artificially by some sort of memorization of the stimuli when they are presented. Muter (1980) conducted an experiment that was similar to the one devised by Peterson and Peterson (1959), except that subjects did not expect to have to recall the consonants. This was arranged through an experimental design in which—when the period after the presentation of the consonants was filled with a second, different task (counting in one experiment, reading words in another)—recall of the consonants usually was not requested. Therefore, whenever the counting or reading task was encountered, recall of the consonants would not be anticipated by the subjects. On rare occasions, though, a cue to recall the consonants did occur two, four, or eight seconds after the beginning of the intervening task. Consonant recall performance in these trials was much poorer than in Peterson and Peterson's (1959) procedure. In other trials—just after the consonants—immediate recall was requested, and recall in these trials was good. Therefore, plotted across delays of zero, two, four, and six seconds, the rate of forgetting was much steeper than in the usual procedure.

The Muter (1980) result has been taken widely to indicate that, as long as precautions are taken to make sure that recall is unexpected, short-term memory is lost much more quickly than was previously believed. However, Healy and Cunningham (1995) cited something important that may seem obvious with the benefit of hindsight. Most of the severe forgetting occurred between test delays of zero and two seconds in Muter's (1980) findings. In the zero-second delay condition, the subject had no way to know whether the distracting task would be presented, and from the subject's point of view the trial often could turn out to be one in which immediate recall was to be requested. In contrast, the appearance of a distracting task indicated to the subject that recall usually would not be requested on that trial. The difference in expectations with a test delay versus without a test delay can account for the severe forgetting function. The rate of forgetting across two to eight seconds looks similar in form to previous studies. Thus, expectations do appear to influence the performance level of short-term recall, but they do not appear to influence the *rate* of forgetting of information from short-term memory. That rate of forgetting seems similar across all of the procedures discussed here. Forgetting at a similar rate can even be observed when one examines memory for syllables of speech that were ignored at the time that they were presented (Cowan, Lichty, & Grove, 1990).

Working memory

A focus on the practical or working functions of short-term memory (Baddeley & Hitch, 1974) led to a reconceptualization of its structure. Baddeley and Hitch, along with subsequent studies reviewed by Baddeley (1986), showed that storing several numbers in memory had only a minimal effect on the ability to carry out comprehension, reasoning, and problem-solving tasks. This finding led to the notion of a separation between the mechanisms of storage and information processing. In the working memory model of Baddeley (1986), information processing was said to be directed by a set of processes termed the *central executive* because it directs processing, along with mechanisms for the passive storage of various kinds of information. Verbal information is said to be held in a passive, phonological storage buffer, whereas visual and spatial information are said to be held in a passive form designated the *visuospatial sketchpad.* The central executive supposedly has some control over what information enters into these passive stores.

For the present purposes, only verbal processing will be discussed. The phonological buffer was said to hold information only temporarily, and a rehearsal process directed by the central executive (but operating semiautomatically once initiated) was said to allow information to be reentered into the buffer, prolonging the total time of its persistence in that buffer. Phonological storage and rehearsal were said to operate together as an *articulatory loop,* allowing the relatively effortless recycling of the list items currently in memory. Baddeley's view is a precursor of the author's view described earlier (Cowan, 1988, 1995). Baddeley's central executive presumably is aligned with the concept of the focus of attention and awareness, and Baddeley's phonological buffer store is similar to the concept of activated information in memory. One clear difference, however, is that Baddeley has thought of the phonological store as speech specific, whereas in the author's view it could be just a special instance of memory activation, and thus could have many properties in common with other types of sensory and semantic memory activation.

One branch of research on working memory, including most of the research by Baddeley and colleagues, has focused primarily on the nature of the articulatory loop. Another branch, including research by several other investigators, has focused on the ramifications of what is essentially the central executive and its active processes. These branches of research will be discussed.

The articulatory loop

A variety of findings led Baddeley (1986) to his view of the structure of working memory. One central finding to be explained was the finding of Baddeley, Thomson, and Buchanan (1975) that a subject's short-term memory performance for a particular set of items is correlated with the rate at which the subject can pronounce those items. This finding, originally with adults, generally has been shown to hold true no matter whether the variation in pronunciation rate is produced through individual differences, age differences, or stimulus differences (e.g., Hulme, Thomson, Muir, & Lawrence, 1984; Naveh-Benjamin & Ayres, 1986; Schweickert & Boruff, 1986). The relation is such that a subject can recall about as many verbal items of a particular type as he or she can pronounce in about two seconds.

Baddeley's (1986) interpretation of the speech–span relation is that it reflects the speed of rehearsal. He assumed that the two-second limit reflects the useful life of information in the phonological storage buffer, unless the information is reactivated through rehearsal. If a subject can rehearse all items within two seconds, then these can be reactivated within the buffer, the storage limit can be evaded, and, therefore, the items can be recalled. The faster the rehearsal process (in items per second), the larger the number of items that can be recalled.

Strengthening this basic account, two studies have shown that this relationship between speed of production and amount of recall holds when examined across ages and when examined within groups of older children and adults of a particular age but not within groups of children as young as 4 years old (Cowan, Keller, et al., 1994; Gathercole, Adams, & Hitch, 1994). This finding probably occurs because verbal rehearsal is very unsophisticated in young children (Flavell, Beach, & Chinsky, 1966) and suggests that the rehearsal loop account may be oversimplified, an observation that will be discussed later.

It is not clear why the two-second estimate for short-term storage is different from the 20- to 30-second estimate offered on the basis of the short-term memory literature, when otherwise they may be assumed to reflect the same storage process. One possibility is that the test conditions make a big difference. The two-second estimate is obtained only in the presence of interference between items; that is, as any one item is rehearsed, it may interfere with the memory representation of other items, and therefore shorten the useful lifetime of the memory. The longer, 20- to 30-second estimate for short-term memory has been obtained in situations without such intense interference or rivalry between items in memory. Perhaps differences in the length of short-term memory demonstrated in various procedures reflect the persistence of memory with versus without interference.

Several other effects and their interaction have served as the mainstays of the articulatory loop account. First, memory for dissimilar-sounding items is better than memory for similar-sounding items. Specifically, in the *phonological similarity effect* (Conrad, 1964), listed items with similar-sounding names (e.g., letters from the set B,C,D,G,P,T,V,Z) are not recalled as well as sets of items with dissimilar names (e.g., letters from the set B,F,J,L,N,Q,R,X). This effect is obtained even when the items are presented visually. This finding suggests that visual representations are used to produce secondary phonological representations. Also, shorter words are usually recalled better than longer words. In this *word length effect* (Baddeley et al., 1975), words that take less time to pronounce are recalled better than words that take longer to pronounce, even if the words classified as "longer" and "shorter" according to this criterion are equated for the number of phonemes and syllables (Baddeley et al., 1975; Cowan et al.,

1992). Finally, speech production can interfere with memory. In the *articulatory suppression effect,* performance is impaired when rehearsal is blocked by the requirement that the subject repeat a word or simple phrase (e.g., "the, the, the") throughout the recall task (Murray, 1968). Interference is greater than in a control task that requires a nonarticulatory type of repetitive motion, such as finger-tapping.

An interpretation of all of these effects (Baddeley, Lewis, & Vallar, 1984) is that they involve several kinds of interference with the operation of the articulatory loop. Phonological similarity effects may occur because phonological similarity makes it difficult to retrieve a particular item from the passive phonological store. In contrast, word length effects may occur because longer words cannot be rehearsed or pronounced as quickly as shorter ones. This difference in mechanisms makes sense because Baddeley et al. (1984) found that articulatory suppression could eliminate the word length effect, but not the phonological similarity effect.

One final effect that was interpreted in terms of the articulatory loop was the effect of irrelevant speech. Salamé and Baddeley (1982) found that irrelevant speech (series of spoken words or a prose passage) did have a large, detrimental effect on a visually presented, verbal short-term recall task that was performed at the same time. Moreover, the effect was larger when the irrelevant speech items were phonologically similar to the items to be recalled. This was taken as evidence that irrelevant speech automatically enters the phonological storage buffer that is used to retain the items to be recalled (in contrast to visual items, which were said to enter only if the appropriate articulatory processing is performed).

Jones and associates have reported a number of studies questioning the basis of the irrelevant speech effect. Jones and Macken (1993) reported that interference with verbal short-term recall also could be obtained with irrelevant, changing tones and suggested that it is the changing state of the irrelevant sounds that produces interference. In fact, Jones, Madden, and Miles (1992) found little effect of irrelevant speech that did not change. Furthermore, contrary to Salamé and Baddeley (1982), Jones and Macken (1995) found little effect of the phonological similarity between the relevant visual and irrelevant spoken items and attributed the finding of Salamé and Baddeley to confounding factors in their stimuli. Tentatively, the findings of Jones and colleagues lend credence to the idea that the phonological storage buffer is not an isolated, specialized module, but rather an integral part of a larger, interactive memory activation system that includes—at the least—nonspeech as well as speech sounds, as suggested by Cowan (1988, 1995).

Research on central executive processes

Baddeley's studies have touched on the central executive and its relation to the articulatory loop and other peripheral systems in various ways (e.g., see Baddeley, 1986). However, a study by Daneman and Carpenter (1980) has been perhaps the most influential in the field. The motivation of the research was that short-term memory spans have been found to bear only weak correlations to intellectual activities such as reasoning, comprehension, and problem solving. Why should this be the case, if short-term memory is used as a working memory that is necessary for these intellectual activities? Daneman and Carpenter suggested that the correlation would be higher for a measure of working memory that required both storage and processing. They developed a *working memory span* measure in which the subject performed two tasks at the same time. Subjects were asked to comprehend sentences and to remember the last word of each sentence. Daneman and Carpenter were interested in the number of sentence–final items that could be recalled under these circumstances. They found that there was a strong correlation between reading comprehension and this working memory span.

The procedure has been applied to many different types of reasoning and comprehension, with positive results (see Ellis Weismer, Chapter 3). Also, Engle and colleagues (e.g., Engle, Cantor, & Carullo, 1992) have found that the procedure is not domain specific. One can use, for example, arithmetic problems and require recall of the final digit from each problem, and this working memory span also correlates with verbal comprehension. What remains unclear is exactly why the procedure works. It may correlate with reasoning and comprehension abilities because—as Daneman and Carpenter assumed—the span measure involves both storage and processing. However, storage of items during a comprehension or calculation task may require an elaborate type of rehearsal, which also may rely heavily on the central executive and not just the articulatory loop. If so, it might be that performance on any difficult dual task would correlate with intellectual skills. Thus, this is an intriguing line of research progress that may well be reinterpreted in the future, in light of future research.

CLINICAL APPLICATIONS TO LANGUAGE

What are the effects of deficits in the central executive and articulatory loop components of Baddeley's model? How does Baddeley's model and other research on the relation between memory impairments and language disabilities provide clinically relevant information?

Deficits in components of Baddeley's model

It is quite clear that intact central executive processes are needed for ordinary thought. Morris (1984, 1986) showed how the contribution of the central executive can be separated from the contribution of the articulatory loop. When patients have damage to the phonological processing centers in the brain, they do not present with the effects that are the hallmark of the phonological loop's contribution to memory, such as the phonological similarity and word length effects. Damage to the central executive appears to lead to a different pattern of memory deficit than damage to the articulatory loop mechanisms. In fact, such damage appears to impair performance on a wide array of cognitive tasks.

The practical importance of the articulatory loop is more subtle. Take, for example, speech comprehension. To comprehend a sentence, one must be able to keep the phonemes in mind at least until they can be converted into words. The neuropsychological literature has suggested that ordinarily phonemes are converted into words quickly. Verbal short-term memory deficits do not translate readily into massive comprehension deficits. However, when a sentence is unusually difficult, if it contains information that must be recalled verbatim, or if it is misleading and must be reinterpreted in the course of listening, then patients with verbal short-term memory deficits experience comprehension difficulties (e.g., Martin, 1993).

Baddeley, Papagno, and Vallar (1988) observed a most interesting patient. Because of a brain lesion, she had a short-term verbal memory span of only a few items. Yet, she functioned successfully as a receptionist and showed no obvious signs of practical inability despite her limited short-term memory span. This case led the investigators to wonder what the use of the articulatory loop actually is—if it is not important for basic comprehension in an ordinary, everyday setting. What they found is that this patient could not learn new vocabulary. She was normal in learning to associate pairs of known words, but she showed virtually no learning when the task was to associate a known word to a new word. The apparent implication is that—to learn a new word—one must hold the phonemic sequence in short-term memory long enough and in enough detail for it to become embedded as a stable lexical unit in long-term memory.

This idea has been applied also to vocabulary acquisition in childhood. Gathercole and Baddeley (1989) used a *nonword repetition* task in which performance was scored on the basis of the length of nonsense words that could be repeated accurately, to eliminate any contribution of the semantic codes that exist for real words. They found that children with a higher nonword repetition score at age 4 had a better vocabulary at age 5. This relation was not symmetrical (i.e., vocabulary at age 4 did not correlate with nonword repetition at age 5). Adams and Gathercole (1995) made the case that this phonological memory impairment also has implications for the syntactic and semantic richness of speech production. However, there is a limited age range for the controlling effects of phonological memory. Gathercole, Willis, Emslie, and Baddeley (1992) found that the relations were different between the ages of 5 and 6. Vocabulary at age 5 predicted nonword repetition at age 6, but nonword repetition at age 5 did not predict vocabulary at age 6.

Gathercole and Baddeley (1990) also showed that nonword repetition was much poorer in children with language impairment (averaging 8.5 years in age) than in either a group of children without language impairment with the same nonverbal ability levels, comparable in age, or a group of younger children with the same verbal ability levels as the children with language impairment. Montgomery (1995) has described consequences of phonological memory impairment, as measured in the nonword repetition task, on sentence comprehension in children with language impairments.

A recent interchange between Gathercole and Baddeley (1995) and Howard and van der Lely (1995) shows that there are, however, important unanswered questions regarding the nonword repetition task. These investigators have used tasks that differ in a number of ways, but one important way is cited by Howard and van der Lely:

> van der Lely and Howard found no difference between children with SLI [specific language impairment] in recall of *lists* of single-syllable nonwords, whereas Gathercole and Baddeley found reduced recall of *single* nonwords, particularly when they are more than two syllables

in length. Clearly, however, these are radically different tasks. The van der Lely and Howard experiment does not require phonological assembly and production of nonwords of more than one syllable [as the Gathercole and Baddeley task does], but does stress the phonological short-term memory system. (p. 468)

Howard and van der Lely (1995) suggested that, rather than memory deficiencies, a phonological *output* process could underlie the deficient nonword repetition abilities of children with language impairments. However, Sussman (1993) suggested that a phonological *input* process might underlie deficient nonword repetition ability. A concomitant result that Gathercole and Baddeley (1990) reported was that children with language impairment had normal-speech sound-discrimination abilities. Sussman replicated this finding but found that the children with language impairment were atypical when the identification of each speech syllable, rather than the discrimination among syllables, was required. Regarding nonword repetition, Sussman (1993) suggested that

a more basic preliminary stage than storage is impaired. That is, the children with language impairments either have difficulty in creating the phonological representation or perhaps in encoding (i.e., linking the acoustic information to its phonological representation). Or, the L.I. children experience a faster decay of the phonological trace causing difficulty in translation into a phonological code. (p. 1296)

The nonword repetition task thus must be viewed with caution, pending more research to assist in its interpretation. However, there is another line of research suggesting that children with language disorders have short-term memory difficulties that may not be specifically phonological in nature. Tallal (1973a, 1973b) found that children with language impairment could reproduce the serial order of fewer tones in a sequence than could children without language impairment. They also had more difficulty in perceiving the order of even two tones when the tones were presented rapidly.

Theoretically, it seems possible that a deficiency in memory for tone order could be secondary to a perceptual deficit in perception of tones at rapid rates. However, in a follow-up study of patients 15 to 20 years of age who had "developmental receptive language disorder," Lincoln, Dickstein, Courchesne, Elmasian, and Tallal (1992) found that these patients continued to display poor memory for sequences, even though they no longer were below normal in handling rapid rates of presentation. Moreover, impaired memory for sequences was not found for another group with atypical language—young adults with autism. Thus, there is reason to suspect that serial order memory impairment may be limited to patients with a specific receptive language disorder.

Gillam, Cowan, and Day (1995) recently obtained results that verify the serial order memory deficit and suggest that it applies to verbal memory. They examined short-term memory for a spoken list of words in 9- to 12-year-old children with language disorders, as well as in a group of children matched to this group in age, and another, younger group matched instead in single-word identification level. Overall, memory performance of children with a specific language impairment was equivalent to that of their younger, reading-matched control subjects. For both groups, however, a deficit was obtained when the list was followed by a final spoken item, termed a *suffix* in the experimental literature, that was not to be recalled. It is consistently found that the presence of a suffix impairs the recall of the last few items in the list (Crowder & Morton, 1969). Such was the case for all children, but the suffix effect was much larger for the children with language impairment. Moreover, their differential deficit was obtained only when the responses were scored for correct serial order.

How would serial order memory play a role in language acquisition? It may be that there are two forms of short-term memory storage and that serial order information is present in only one of them, which also happens to be important for language acquisition. A serial order–free form of storage may consist of separate activation processes for long-term memory units corresponding to recently presented items. That sort of memory might not be particularly useful in learning language. A second kind of short-term memory storage may consist of an *overall* pattern of activation that includes the serial order links among recently presented items; perhaps it is prominent only for items presented in the auditory modality. This type of memory could underlie vocabulary acquisition and other aspects of language learning, which involve a great deal of serial order information.

It should be noted that—even if there are problems with Gathercole and Baddeley's (1989, 1990) nonword repetition task, and perhaps with Baddeley's (1986) implication that phonological short-term memory is a speech-specific module—these investigators have been in the right "ballpark" in arguing that short-term memory deficits may play an integral role in language impairments.

RECENT THEORETICAL DEVELOPMENTS AND THEIR IMPLICATIONS

A fairly (if not completely) tidy picture of the current state of understanding has been presented. A brief consideration of four ongoing issues will illustrate that the field and its practical implications are not yet so tidy.

Issue 1: What is the role of speech production in short-term memory?

Recall that Baddeley (1986) observed a rather strong relationship between the rate of speech and short-term recall. One instance of this relationship was the word length effect. Baddeley assumed that the word length effect occurs because longer words take more time to rehearse than shorter words. However, Cowan et al. (1992) found that this is not the only factor. In a short-term recall task with a spoken response, they included mixed lists that began with either short or long words and, independently, ended with either short or long words. They also examined both forward and backward recall. They found that it was the length of words to be recalled first that made the most difference. Presumably, while these words were being pronounced by the subject, the remaining words were being lost from short-term memory. Henry (1991) showed that the effect of memory loss during spoken recall is important in the development of memory. When a nonverbal, pointing response was used, 5-year-old children no longer displayed a word length effect at all, although 7-year-old children still did (presumably because of the contribution of rehearsal).

The degree of importance of speech production for the normal pattern of short-term memory results is still unclear. On one hand, Raine, Hulme, Chadderton, and Bailey (1991) found no evidence of the word length effect in a task using a nonverbal response in children 4 to 15 years old who had slowed speech for a variety of reasons (including a large subgroup of children with dysarthria). On the other hand, Bishop and Robson (1989) found normal word length and phonological similarity effects in a similar task administered (using eye-tracking) to subjects 10 to 18 years old who were congenitally anarthric or dysarthric because of cerebral palsy. It is not yet clear why the results of these studies differ.

The role of speech production must be considered when one is interpreting the literature on memory and language impairments. Consider one example. Kirchner and Klatzky (1985) found a poorer-than-normal quality of rehearsal in children with language impairment who were 7 to 13 years old. They wondered whether rehearsal led to a phonological memory deficit or, conversely, whether it was a fundamental phonological memory deficit that made rehearsal difficult. Gathercole and Baddeley (1990) suggested that the latter was the case, largely because children with language impairment produced a normal-sized word length effect, which suggested that normal rehearsal was happening. However, if one considers that the word length effect could have resulted from memory loss during the spoken response period rather than during rehearsal, then the quality of rehearsal still could be pathological in these children.

Caplan, Rochon, and Waters (1992) had a different explanation for the word length effect. They argued that the effect occurs only because the longer words are phonologically more complex, and they made the effect disappear by equating the complexity of short and long words. However, they used a nonverbal, pointing response in their experiments. Phonological complexity may explain the rehearsal basis of the word length effect (although Baddeley & Andrade, 1994, argued otherwise), but if a spoken response were used, the word length effect might well be obtained even with phonological complexity equated.

An implication of the loss of memory during speaking is that a slowed rate of speech in some individuals with language disorders potentially may make a difference for more complex aspects of their language production. Planned syntactic, semantic, or phonemic information might be lost more quickly during the longer, and perhaps more attention-demanding, speech process in those patients, compared with subjects without language disorders.

Issue 2: What is the role of knowledge retrieval in short-term recall?

Hulme, Maughan, and Brown (1991) showed that the articulatory loop model has merit but is incomplete. They examined adults' memory and rate of speech for sets of short, medium, and long words and nonwords. A graph of the mean speech rate for each condition as a function of the memory span for that condition was linear in form for both words and nonwords, as predicted by the articulatory loop model. However, unlike the model's predictions, the line was higher for the recall of words than for nonwords. This finding indicates that lexical knowledge contributes to recall in a way that is not predicted by the rate of speech of the recordings.

Snowling, Chiat, and Hulme (1991) criticized Gathercole and Baddeley's (1989, 1990) nonword repetition task on the grounds that the application of lexical knowledge to nonwords might help one to repeat them, which would make knowledge—rather than memory per se—the ultimate source of nonword repetition deficits in children with language impairments. However, some recent findings of Gathercole (1995) help to allay these concerns. She separated nonwords into those judged more versus less "wordlike" and found that repetition of the less wordlike nonwords—but not the more wordlike nonwords—at 4 years of age predicted vocabulary scores at ages 4 and 5, as well as reading scores at age 5. Thus, although it does seem that knowledge influences short-term memory, it does not seem to account for individual differences in vocabulary and reading acquisition at this young age.

Issue 3: What is the role of short-term memory search?

It is important to realize that there are many mechanisms involved in a short-term memory task that are outside of the scope of the articulatory loop model. One of these mechanisms is the mental search of short-term memory representations for retrieval of information about the presented list. The existence of a rapid, orderly short-term memory search was first demonstrated by Sternberg (1966). On each trial within his procedure, a short list of one to six items was presented and then a "probe item" was presented. The task was to indicate—as quickly as possible—whether the probe item did or did not appear in the immediately preceding list. The time it took to indicate this increased steadily as the number of items in the list increased. However, the search appeared to be quite rapid in that the extra search time increased only about 40 milliseconds for each additional list item. In children, the search process can take more than five times as long (e.g., Keating, Keniston, Manis, & Bobbitt, 1980).

The procedure used in the search task is quite different from the ordinary short-term memory procedure, but there are reasons to suspect that a similar process applies. In particular, the speed at which a subject can determine which item to recall next during a serial recall trial may depend on how quickly that subject can search through the mental representation of the list.

Strengthening this hypothesis, Cavanagh (1972) found a strong linear relation between the mean serial recall for a particular type of list (consonants, digits, etc.) and the mean memory search rate in Sternberg's type of procedure for the same type of list. Puckett and Kausler (1984) found the same thing using within-subject measures of the correlation. A relevance of this correlation to individual differences is suggested by the finding of Sininger, Klatzky, and Kirchner (1989) of impaired memory search in children with language impairments.

Memory search may be important within the response phase of list recall trials because the faster the memory search, the shorter the period during which items potentially could be lost from the short-term memory representation through temporal decay or interference. The author has examined one direct index of short-term retrieval in a serial recall task: the mean duration of the silent pauses between words in the responses within spoken recall. Specifically, in a study of spoken recall in 4-year-olds, Cowan (1992) found that interword pauses in the responses increased with list length and, for a particular list length, were shorter for children with higher memory spans. Cowan, Wood, and Borne (1994) found that, for a particular list length, 8-year-old children had shorter interword pauses than 4-year-old children. It will be interesting to determine whether memory search in the memory span task, reflected in these interword pause times, correlates well with memory search in Sternberg's probe procedure. This basic short-term memory search procedure may have to be added to theories of verbal memory span for performance to be understood adequately.

An unanswered question is how much the speed of the search process really is distinct from another speed involved in memory span—namely the speed of verbal rehearsal. Kail and Park (1994) suggested that verbal rehearsal is one manifestation of an individual's overall, global processing speed, and according to their approach it might be expected that memory search speed would be another manifestation of global speed. Contrary to this expectation, however, Cowan, Wood, and Keller (1995) found that memory search speeds and speaking rates were not correlated with one another, although both were correlated with memory span. Search rate and speaking rate together accounted for 60% of the variance in memory span within a developmental study. The factors contributing to short-term memory performance are not extremely simple, but researchers, and consequently clinicians, are beginning to gain a better understanding of them.

Issue 4: Is there clear evidence for a separate short-term memory mechanism?

The most provocative unresolved question also is the oldest. Not everyone believes in a separate short-term memory mechanism. Instead, some researchers hope that any sort of memory process, long or short—from retaining a phone number to recalling a memorized passage from a play—could be accounted for through a common set of learning and memory principles.

Procedures showing that memory in the short term differs from memory in the longer term have been presented. Across relatively long postlist test delays, for example, subjects lose the recency effect, the special advantage that ordinarily occurs for the recall of items at the end of a verbal list (Glanzer & Cunitz, 1966). However, it had been assumed but not demonstrated that this effect of test delay occurred because the amount of forgetting increased with the amount of time during which the information had to be retained. Instead, some subsequent research has suggested that it is the *relative* amount of time that is critical, not the absolute amount.

Bjork and Whitten (1974) found recency effects when periods filled with a distracting task—12 to 20 seconds in duration—were introduced between pairs of items and at the end of the list. Under these circumstances, there was a strong recency effect in the free recall of the words, despite the long test delay. If the absolute passage of time were especially critical for recall, the recency effect should have disappeared across the list-final period. An alternative explanation is that the recency effect occurs because the passage of time removes the distinctiveness of the list-final items. When one recalls immediately, the time since the last item is small compared with the time since the prior items; therefore, the last item seems distinct. However, when one recalls after a distractor-filled period, the time since the last list item seems similar to the time since the prior items, removing that distinctiveness of the last item. Other research has shown that the modality and suffix effects also can be obtained with this type of procedure in which items are separated by distractor periods (e.g., Glenberg, 1984). The basis of recall in the Peterson and Peterson (1959) procedure has been challenged on similar grounds (e.g., Crowder, 1993).

Cowan (1988, 1995) argued that there are subtle but important differences in the findings for the recall of ordinary versus distractor-separated lists. Perhaps the most straightforward example is the finding of Cowan, Wood, and Borne (1994). They found that, although the recency advantage was obtained when lists were separated by distractor periods, under these conditions the word length effect was not obtained. Thus, although some short-term memory phenomena (e.g., the recency effect) will have to be reinterpreted, there are other phenomena that appear to confirm the need to postulate a separate short-term memory mechanism that truly is preserved in the brain for only a fixed, brief period of time. However, we cannot yet be sure.

•   •   •

In summary, this chapter has examined the basic mechanisms of short-term and working memory, the recent applications of the concepts emerging from research with clinical populations, and unresolved theoretical issues in the field. The research on basic mechanisms in individuals without language disorders points out factors of importance in recalling recently encountered information, such as the phonological system, articulatory processes used to rehearse stored verbal information, and attentive and effortful (central executive) mental processes used to direct memory storage and retrieval.

The clinical applications suggest that intact phonological short-term memory and articulatory processes are important in language acquisition and that all of the components of working memory—operating together—are important in a wide array of mental tasks such as comprehension, reasoning, and problem solving. The recent research suggests that additional processes and factors that were not included in traditional models of short-term memory may make an important difference in short-term recall. These factors include the spoken versus nonspoken mode in which information is requested from subjects or patients, the subjects' or patients' knowledge and familiarity with the materials, and their ability to search rapidly through the memory representation.

Even the special nature of short-term memory storage, as opposed to memory in general, has been questioned. If it turns out (against the odds, the author believes) that there is only one set of principles for all of learning and memory regardless of the time scales, then, paradoxically, the author still would not be convinced that the chapter has been presented in vain. Children and other individuals with language disorders show a distinct pattern of deficits on short-term memory tasks and that is likely to be important no matter what the combination of receptive, storage, and productive processes that explains the pattern.

REFERENCES

Adams, A.M., & Gathercole, S.E. (1995). Phonological working memory and speech production in preschool children. *Journal of Speech and Hearing Research, 38*, 403–414.

Baddeley, A.D. (1986). *Working memory.* Oxford, England: Clarendon Press.

Baddeley, A., & Andrade, J. (1994). Reversing the word-length effect: A comment on Caplan, Rochon, and Waters. *Quarterly Journal of Experimental Psychology, 47A,* 1047–1054.

Baddeley, A., & Hitch, G.J. (1974). Working memory. In G. Bower (Ed.), *The psychology of learning and motivation* (Vol. 8). New York: Academic Press.

Baddeley, A., Lewis, V., & Vallar, G. (1984). Exploring the articulatory loop. *Quarterly Journal of Experimental Psychology, 36A,* 233–252.

Baddeley, A., Papagno, C., & Vallar, G. (1988). When long-term learning depends on short-term storage. *Journal of Memory and Language, 27,* 586–595.

Baddeley, A.D., Thomson, N., & Buchanan, M. (1975). Word length and the structure of short-term memory. *Journal of Verbal Learning and Verbal Behavior, 14,* 575–589.

Balota, D.A. (1983). Automatic semantic activation and episodic memory encoding. *Journal of Verbal Learning and Verbal Behavior, 22,* 88–104.

Bentin, S., Kutas, M., & Hillyard, S.A. (1995). Semantic processing and memory for attended and unattended words in dichotic listening: Behavioral and electrophysiological evidence. *Journal of Experimental Psychology: Human Perception and Performance, 21,* 54–67.

Bishop, D.V.M., & Robson, J. (1989). Unimpaired short-term memory and rhyme judgment in congenitally speechless individuals: Implications for the notion of "articulatory coding." *Quarterly Journal of Experimental Psychology, 41A,* 123–140.

Bjork, R.A., & Whitten, W.B. (1974). Recency-sensitive retrieval processes in long-term free recall. *Cognitive Psychology, 6,* 173–189.

Caplan, D., Rochon, E., & Waters, G.S. (1992). Articulatory and phonological determinants of word length effects in span tasks. *Quarterly Journal of Experimental Psychology, 45A,* 177–192.

Cavanagh, J.P. (1972). Relation between the immediate memory span and the memory search rate. *Psychological Review, 79,* 525–530.

Conrad, R. (1964). Acoustic confusion in immediate memory. *British Journal of Psychology, 55,* 75–84.

Cowan, N. (1988). Evolving conceptions of memory storage, selective attention, and their mutual constraints within the human information processing system. *Psychological Bulletin, 104,* 163–191.

Cowan, N. (1992). Verbal memory span and the timing of spoken recall. *Journal of Memory and Language, 31,* 668–684.

Cowan, N. (1995). *Attention and memory: An integrated framework.* New York: Oxford University Press.

Cowan, N., Day, L., Saults, J.S., Keller, T.A., Johnson, T., & Flores, L. (1992). The role of verbal output time in the effects of word length on immediate memory. *Journal of Memory and Language, 31*, 1–17.

Cowan, N., Keller, T., Hulme, C., Roodenrys, S., McDougall, S., & Rack, J. (1994). Verbal memory span in children: Speech timing clues to the mechanisms underlying age and word length effects. *Journal of Memory and Language, 33*, 234–250.

Cowan, N., Lichty, W., & Grove, T.R. (1990). Properties of memory for unattended spoken syllables. *Journal of Experimental Psychology: Learning, Memory, and Cognition, 16*, 258–269.

Cowan, N., Wood, N.L., & Borne, D.N. (1994). Reconfirmation of the short-term storage concept. *Psychological Science, 5*, 103–106.

Cowan, N., Wood, N., & Keller, T. (1995, April). *Why is speaking rate correlated with memory span?* Paper presented at the biennial convention of the Society for Research in Child Development, Indianapolis, IN.

Crowder, R.G. (1993). Short-term memory: Where do we stand? *Memory and Cognition, 21*, 142–145.

Crowder, R.G., & Morton, J. (1969). Precategorical acoustic storage. *Perception and Psychophysics, 5*, 365–373.

Daneman, M., & Carpenter, P.A. (1980). Individual differences in working memory and reading. *Journal of Verbal Learning and Verbal Behavior, 19*, 450–466.

Engle, R.W., Cantor, J., & Carullo, J.J. (1992). Individual differences in working memory and comprehension: A test of four hypotheses. *Journal of Experimental Psychology: Learning, Memory, and Cognition, 18*, 972–992.

Flavell, J.H., Beach, D.H., & Chinsky, J.M. (1966). Spontaneous verbal rehearsal in a memory task as a function of age. *Child Development, 37*, 283–299.

Gathercole, S.E. (1995). Is nonword repetition a test of phonological memory or long-term knowledge? It all depends on the nonwords. *Memory and Cognition, 23*, 83–94.

Gathercole, S.E., Adams, A.-M., & Hitch, G.J. (1994). Do young children rehearse? An individual-differences analysis. *Memory and Cognition, 22*, 201–207.

Gathercole, S.E., & Baddeley, A.D. (1989). Evaluation of the role of phonological STM in the development of vocabulary in children: A longitudinal study. *Journal of Memory and Language, 28*, 200–213.

Gathercole, S.E., & Baddeley, A. (1990). Phonological memory deficits in language disordered children: Is there a causal connection? *Journal of Memory and Language, 29*, 336–360.

Gathercole, S.E., & Baddeley, A. (1995). Short-term memory may yet be deficient in children with language impairments: A comment on van der Lely & Howard (1993). *Journal of Speech and Hearing Research, 38*, 463–466.

Gathercole, S.E., Willis, C., Emslie, H., & Baddeley, A. (1992). Phonological memory and vocabulary development during the early school years: A longitudinal study. *Developmental Psychology, 28*, 887–898.

Gillam, R.B., Cowan, N., & Day, L.S. (1995). Sequential memory in children with and without language impairment. *Journal of Speech and Hearing Research, 38,* 393–402.

Glanzer, M., & Cunitz, A.R. (1966). Two storage mechanisms in free recall. *Journal of Verbal Learning and Verbal Behavior, 5,* 351–360.

Glenberg, A.M. (1984). A retrieval account of the long-term modality effect. *Journal of Experimental Psychology: Learning, Memory, and Cognition, 10,* 16–31.

Healy, A.F., & Cunningham, T.F. (1995). Very rapid forgetting: Reply to Muter. *Memory and Cognition, 23,* 387–392.

Hebb, D.O. (1949). *Organization of behavior.* New York: Wiley.

Henry, L.A. (1991). The effects of word length and phonemic similarity in young children's short-term memory. *Quarterly Journal of Experimental Psychology, 43A,* 35–52.

Holender, D. (1986). Semantic activation without conscious identification in dichotic listening, parafoveal vision, and visual masking: A survey and appraisal. *Behavioral and Brain Sciences, 9,* 1–66.

Howard, D., & van der Lely, H.K.J. (1995). Specific language impairment in children is *not* due to a short-term memory deficit: Response to Gathercole and Baddeley. *Journal of Speech and Hearing Research, 38,* 466–472.

Hulme, C., Maughan, S., & Brown, G.D.A. (1991). Memory for familiar and unfamiliar words: Evidence for a long-term memory contribution to short-term memory span. *Journal of Memory and Language, 30,* 685–701.

Hulme, C., Thomson, N., Muir, C., & Lawrence, A. (1984). Speech rate and the development of short-term memory span. *Journal of Experimental Child Psychology, 38,* 241–253.

James, W. (1890). *The principles of psychology.* New York: Henry Holt.

Jones, D.M., & Macken, W.J. (1993). Irrelevant tones produce an "irrelevant speech effect": Implications for phonological coding in working memory. *Journal of Experimental Psychology: Learning, Memory, and Cognition, 19,* 369–381.

Jones, D.M., & Macken, W.J. (1995). Phonological similarity in the irrelevant speech effect: Within- or between-stream similarity? *Journal of Experimental Psychology: Learning, Memory, and Cognition, 21,* 103–115.

Jones, D.M., Madden, C., & Miles, C. (1992). Privileged access by irrelevant speech to short-term memory: The role of changing state. *Quarterly Journal of Experimental Psychology, 44A,* 645–669.

Kail, R., & Park, Y.-S. (1994). Processing time, articulation time, and memory span. *Journal of Experimental Child Psychology, 57,* 281–291.

Keating, D.P., Keniston, A.H., Manis, F.R., & Bobbitt, B.L. (1980). Development of the search-processing parameter. *Child Development, 51,* 39–44.

Kirchner, D.M., & Klatzky, R.L. (1985). Verbal rehearsal and memory in language-disordered children. *Journal of Speech and Hearing Research, 28,* 556–565.

Lincoln, A.J., Dickstein, P., Courchesne, E., Elmasian, R., & Tallal, P. (1992). Auditory processing abilities in non-retarded adolescents and young adults with developmental receptive language disorder and autism. *Brain and Language, 43,* 613–622.

Marcel, A.J. (1983). Conscious and unconscious perception: Experiments on visual masking and word recognition. *Cognitive Psychology, 15,* 197–237.

Martin, R.C. (1993). Short-term memory and sentence processing: Evidence from neuropsychology. *Memory and Cognition, 21,* 176–183.

Miller, G.A. (1956). The magical number seven, plus or minus two: Some limits on our capacity for processing information. *Psychological Review, 63,* 81–97.

Montgomery, J.W. (1995). Sentence comprehension in children with specific language impairment: The role of phonological working memory. *Journal of Speech and Hearing Research, 38,* 187–199.

Moray, N. (1959). Attention in dichotic listening: Affective cues and the influence of instructions. *Quarterly Journal of Experimental Psychology, 11,* 56–60.

Morris, R.G. (1984). Dementia and the functioning of the articulatory loop system. *Cognitive Neuropsychology, 1,* 143–158.

Morris, R.G. (1986). Short term memory in senile dementia of the Alzheimer's type. *Cognitive Neuropsychology, 3,* 77–97.

Murray, D.J. (1968). Articulation and acoustic confusability in short-term memory. *Journal of Experimental Psychology, 78,* 679–684.

Muter, P. (1980). Very rapid forgetting. *Memory and Cognition, 8,* 174–179.

Naveh-Benjamin, M., & Ayres, T.J. (1986). Digit span, reading rate, and linguistic relativity. *Quarterly Journal of Experimental Psychology, 38A,* 739–751.

Peterson, L.R., & Peterson, M.J. (1959). Short-term retention of individual verbal items. *Journal of Experimental Psychology, 58,* 193–198.

Puckett, J.M., & Kausler, D.H. (1984). Individual differences and models of memory span: A role for memory search rate? *Journal of Experimental Psychology: Learning, Memory, and Cognition, 10,* 72–82.

Raine, A., Hulme, C., Chadderton, H., & Bailey, P. (1991). Verbal short-term memory span in speech-disordered children: Implications for articulatory coding in short-term memory. *Child Development, 62,* 415–423.

Sachs, J.S. (1967). Recognition memory for syntactic and semantic aspects of connected discourse. *Perception and Psychophysics, 2,* 437–442.

Salamé, P., & Baddeley, A. (1982). Disruption of short-term memory by unattended speech: Implications for the structure of working memory. *Journal of Verbal Learning and Verbal Behavior, 21,* 150–164.

Schweickert, R., & Boruff, B. (1986). Short-term memory capacity: Magic number or magic spell? *Journal of Experimental Psychology: Learning, Memory, and Cognition, 12,* 419–425.

Sininger, Y.S., Klatzky, R.L., & Kirchner, D.M. (1989). Memory scanning speed in language-disordered children. *Journal of Speech and Hearing Research, 32,* 289–297.

Snowling, M., Chiat, S., & Hulme, C. (1991). Words, non-words and phonological processes: Some comments on Gathercole, Willis, Emslie, and Baddeley. *Applied Psycholinguistics, 12,* 369–373.

Sternberg, S. (1966). High-speed scanning in human memory. *Science, 153*, 652–654.

Sussman, J.E. (1993). Perception of formant transition cues to place of articulation in children with language impairments. *Journal of Speech and Hearing Research, 36*, 1286–1299.

Tallal, P. (1973a). Defects of non-verbal auditory perception in children with developmental aphasia. *Nature, 241*, 468–469.

Tallal, P. (1973b). Developmental aphasia: Impaired rate of nonverbal processing as a function of sensory modality. *Neuropsychologia, 11*, 389–398.

Wood, N., & Cowan, N. (1995). The cocktail party phenomenon revisited: How frequent are attention shifts to one's name in an irrelevant auditory channel? *Journal of Experimental Psychology: Learning, Memory, and Cognition, 21*, 255–260.

2

Sentence Comprehension and Working Memory in Children with Specific Language Impairment

James W. Montgomery

Seven-year-old Nicholas was leaving the examining room when an examiner reminded him, "Before you go to lunch, don't forget to get your coat that's hanging on the coatrack in the waiting room." Nicholas smiled, politely shook his head, and immediately looked at his mother, apparently for assistance. A linguistic encounter such as this is a part of everyday conversation and presents little or no difficulty for children without language disabilities, but for Nicholas and many other children with specific language impairment (SLI) such encounters are anything but routine. If not on a primarily linguistic basis, how might such apparent language understanding difficulties in these children be accounted for? It will be argued here that a profitable way of explaining some of the comprehension difficulties exhibited by some children with SLI is to consider language processing (comprehension, in this case) as being influenced by a limited-capacity working memory system (e.g., Baddeley, 1986; Carpenter, Just, & Shell, 1990; Lahey & Bloom, 1994). The case will be made that in some children with SLI, difficulties understanding sentences may be related to how well they manage their more-limited working memory resources.

It is not unreasonable to think that the sentence comprehension of some children with SLI might be hampered at times by a limitation in memory functioning. A number of researchers, in fact, have made the claim that the

Top Lang Disord 1996;17(1):19–32
© 1996 Aspen Publishers, Inc.

language impairment of many children with SLI may be related in part to some sort of memory deficit (e.g., Ceci, Ringstrom, & Lea, 1981; Curtiss & Tallal, 1991; Graham, 1980). Indeed, children with SLI may exhibit a variety of verbal short-term memory (STM) deficits, including retaining sequential order of information (Gillam, Cowan, & Day, 1995), the rate at which they scan STM for verbal information (Sininger, Klatzky, & Kirchner, 1989), retrieving words from word lists (Ceci et al., 1981; Kail, Hale, Leonard, & Nippold, 1984), recalling information from stories (Graybeal, 1981), and reduced verbal capacity (Gathercole & Baddeley, 1990a; Kirchner & Klatzky, 1985; Montgomery, 1995a).

Importantly, although evidence of various STM difficulties in these children grows, the nature of any potential relation between their verbal STM and sentence comprehension difficulties has yet to be established. Recently, Curtiss and Tallal (1991) have argued, based on indirect evidence, that the poor sentence-level syntactic comprehension of some children with SLI stems not from a lack of linguistic knowledge but more from a limitation in STM. They compared the influence of syntactic redundancy (i.e., long versus short sentences of comparable syntactic structure and meaning) on the sentence comprehension of children with SLI and two groups of developing children without SLI. The children heard nonredundant sentences of the sort "The girl smiling is pushing the boy laughing" and redundant sentences such as "The girl who is smiling is pushing the boy who is laughing." The age-matched control subjects "preferred" the redundant sentences, as did the language-matched control subjects when they got older. However, the children with SLI (regardless of age) "preferred" the shorter, nonredundant sentences. These authors, then, proposed that an impairment in verbal STM was responsible for the poorer processing of the redundant, longer sentences by the children with SLI. Although these results certainly hint at the possibility of some kind of link between STM and sentence comprehension difficulties in children with SLI, this study was not designed to identify which specific verbal STM process(es) might undermine these children's comprehension efforts. From a clinical point of view, many speech-language pathologists (SLPs) also seem to have an impression that some of the sentence comprehension difficulties of some children with SLI seem to be related to an STM problem. The all-important clinical question is in what way(s) might these two difficulties relate.

A MODEL OF WORKING MEMORY

Many researchers have argued that complex cognition such as language comprehension (Just & Carpenter, 1992; Kintsch & Van Dijk, 1978), reasoning (Carpenter, Just, & Shell, 1990), and academic achievement (Engle, Cantor, & Carullo, 1992) is mediated to some extent by a limited-capacity mechanism referred to as *working memory* (WM). A number of models of WM have been proposed (e.g., Baddeley, 1986; Just & Carpenter, 1992; Kintsch & Van Dijk, 1978). All differ in important—sometimes subtle—ways regarding their structural and functional characteristics. It should be noted, however, that with respect to sentence comprehension there are some researchers who argue that WM plays little or no role at all (e.g., Butterworth, Campbell, & Howard, 1986; Martin, 1987).

A substantial body of research suggests a strong association between WM and sentence comprehension. In adult readers, for example, King and Just (1991) found that those college students with low WM capacity demonstrated poorer syntactic processing than "high-capacity" students. Similarly, Daneman and Carpenter (1983) have shown that poor comprehension on certain reading tasks in college students can be predicted by individual differences in WM capacity. Bar-Shalom, Crain, and Shankweiler (1993) also have argued—based on their data—that the poorer syntactic comprehension of many school-age children with reading problems is caused by a WM capacity limitation. Baddeley and colleagues (e.g., Baddeley, Vallar, & Wilson, 1987; Vallar & Baddeley, 1984) have shown that poor auditory sentence comprehension of adults with brain injury is strongly associated with limited WM capacity. From a developmental language perspective, Gathercole and associates (Gathercole & Baddeley, 1990b; Gathercole, Willis, Emslie, & Baddeley, 1992) have reported that phonological WM capacity and vocabulary growth are highly correlated in 4- to 6-year-old, developing children without language disorders. They showed that children with "low" phonological WM capacity develop less extensive vocabularies than children with "high" capacity. Finally, Adams and Gathercole (1995) have reported a strong association between WM capacity and very young children's ability to produce multiword utterances. In short, a variety of linguistic skills have been shown to be strongly associated with WM.

Although Cowan (Chapter 1) presents a thorough overview of the construct of WM and how it differs from a more conventional concept of

STM, in this chapter the focus is on one particular model of WM. The model advanced by Baddeley and colleagues (Baddeley & Hitch, 1974; Baddeley et al., 1987; Gathercole & Baddeley, 1993; Vallar & Baddeley, 1984) will be presented, and the focus will be on how it seems to relate to the process of sentence comprehension. Baddeley's model has proved powerful in detailing the role that WM seems to play in sentence comprehension in unimpaired and impaired adult listeners. The power of Baddeley's model derives from its clear delineation of how the articulatory loop system of WM (see Cowan, Chapter 1) seems to be involved in sentence comprehension. For this reason, Baddeley's model appears to be well suited for examining the nature of the association between "STM" (WM specifically) and auditory sentence comprehension difficulties in children with SLI.

Baddeley's concept of the articulatory loop, which has received considerable research attention and empirical support, is specialized for the short-term maintenance and processing of linguistic material. The articulatory loop is made up of two components: a phonological short-term store and an articulatory control process (i.e., articulatory rehearsal). The phonological store represents and retains speech material in the form of a phonological code. This representation decays rapidly with time. Articulatory rehearsal functions to refresh and maintain linguistic material in the store (via subvocal or overt rehearsal) before it decays. Spoken input enters the phonological store directly, without the need for rehearsal. Because most spoken language comprehension occurs in real time whereby listeners construct sentence meaning immediately (Marslen-Wilson & Tyler, 1980; Marslen-Wilson & Welsh, 1978), the phonological loop presumably is not needed. That is, because comprehension develops immediately, there is no need for the listener to retain and refresh a phonological record of the input in the phonological store. However, for sentences that are complex in structure (e.g., "The boy that was kissed by the girl fell off the bench") or lengthy (e.g., "Put the vegetables and meat in the bins and the bananas and peaches in the basket hanging by the window"), or when the preservation of word order is critical to sentence interpretation (e.g., "It was John not Larry who took Jim's wallet"), a phonological record of the input (or a portion of it) presumably is needed. This record is "consulted" or reanalyzed and interpreted, thus increasing the likelihood that the input will be comprehended (Baddeley, 1986). The phonological record may be refreshed via articulatory rehearsal, depending on its length. In essence, the phonological store component of the loop functions much like a mnemonic window in which sequences of incoming words are held in serial order while the items within the sequences are processed and interpreted. Like the central executive, the phonological store has limited capacity. If the amount of speech material exceeds a listener's capacity, comprehension will suffer. In short, then, successful language understanding depends on the continuous and immediate integration of information in WM, requiring listeners to simultaneously store and process verbal information.

The operations of WM in sentence comprehension can be illustrated with the following example of a direction that might be heard by a school-age child in the classroom: "Turn in the math problems that you completed on page 43, then begin working only on the division problems on page 51." One scenario for processing and comprehending this command might be that the first two clauses of the sentence ("Turn in the math problems that you completed on page 43") will be stored in the central executive after they have been processed for meaning. Although the phonological loop is free of information (given that the first half of the command resides in the central executive), the second part of the command ("then begin working only on the division problems on page 51") enters the loop, where it is temporarily held long enough (perhaps refreshed via rehearsal) to be ana-lyzed and interpreted. When this part of the command has been interpreted, it is subsequently integrated with the first half of the command in the cen-tral executive. For most developing children without language disorders, such input is comprehended fairly easily. However, for some children with SLI, such input may be difficult to comprehend because of an inefficiency managing the operations of WM—the central executive and/or the phono-logical loop. Research with adults and children with language and/or read-ing disabilities has shown that difficulty managing either the central ex-ecutive (e.g., Oakhill, Yuill, & Parkin, 1988; Yuill, Oakhill, & Parkin, 1989) or the phonological loop (e.g., Baddeley et al., 1987; Vallar & Baddeley, 1984) is strongly associated with poor auditory and reading comprehension.

WORKING MEMORY AND SENTENCE COMPREHENSION IN CHILDREN WITH SLI

Although WM has not been investigated extensively in children with SLI, studies have focused on the phonological loop and generally have yielded consistent results and interpretations (Gathercole & Baddeley,

1990a; James, van Steenbrugge, & Chiveralls, 1994; Montgomery, 1995a; however, see van der Lely & Howard, 1993, for a different interpretation regarding a capacity deficit). Gathercole and Baddeley (1990a) showed, for the first time, that the phonological store component of the loop in children with SLI is reduced in capacity. They used a nonsense word repetition task to assess their subjects' phonological memory capacity. Their subjects with SLI had significant difficulties repeating three-syllable and four-syllable nonsense words relative to one- and two-syllable nonsense words. Given this response pattern (i.e., word length effect) by the children with SLI, Gathercole and Baddeley argued that these children had reduced phonological memory capacity, resulting in their storing less phonological information than the control children.

Only one study has examined the association between phonological WM and sentence-level comprehension abilities in children with SLI (Montgomery, 1995b). The study was designed in part to replicate the findings of Gathercole and Baddeley (1990a) indicating that children with SLI have a limitation in phonological memory capacity and the findings of Curtiss and Tallal (1991) showing that children with SLI have more trouble processing longer, linguistically redundant sentences than shorter, nonredundant sentences. The key question of the study, however, was whether subjects' performance on the phonological WM task and the sentence comprehension task would be positively correlated. Performance on a nonsense word repetition task served as the index of phonological WM capacity. In the sentence comprehension task, 14 children with SLI and 13 children without SLI matched on sentence-level comprehension abilities listened to sentences that were linguistically redundant or nonredundant. The two sentence types were nearly structurally identical and encoded essentially the same semantic information. The only difference between the sentence types was that the linguistic cues and the modifying adjectival/adverbial words in the redundant sentences were absent in the nonredundant sentences, thus making the nonredundant sentences shorter (e.g., "Point to the picture of the cats" versus "Point to the picture of the two cats," "The little boy standing is hitting the little girl sitting" versus "The little boy who is standing is hitting the little girl who is sitting"). After listening to a tape-recorded sentence, subjects selected from an array of pictures the one corresponding to what they had heard.

The results of the nonsense word repetition task were clear-cut. As already mentioned, the children with SLI repeated significantly fewer three-

and four-syllable items than one- and two-syllable items relative to themselves and their peers, suggesting that they had reduced phonological WM capacity. The results of the sentence comprehension task also were clearcut. Whereas the children without SLI comprehended equal numbers of redundant and nonredundant sentences, the children with SLI comprehended significantly fewer of the redundant sentences than the nonredundant sentences. Also, compared with their peers, the children with SLI were found to comprehend fewer of the redundant sentences but a comparable number of nonredundant sentences.

To examine the relation between phonological WM capacity and sentence comprehension, the investigators computed a Pearson product–moment correlation for nonsense word repetition performance and performance on the sentence comprehension task. A positive correlation was found ($r = .62, p < .001$). A scatterplot of individual subject's performances on each task clearly indicated that those children who performed poorly on the repetition task also performed poorly on the sentence comprehension task (i.e., children with SLI). Conversely, those who did well on the repetition task also did well on the comprehension task (i.e., control children). On the whole, the findings were interpreted to suggest that, relative to their peers without SLI, the children with SLI comprehended fewer longer sentences because they had more limited phonological WM capacity and thus were less able to hold as much verbal material in their phonological store.

Although it is tempting to say that a limitation in phonological WM capacity may be a prime culprit in the comprehension problems of some children with SLI, this limitation may be only part of the picture. It is important to consider that the central executive also may be deficient in children with SLI. These children may have trouble managing and coordinating the regulatory functions of the central executive (e.g., making decisions about how to simultaneously direct and allocate resources to different portions of the input or to different cognitive functions) and/or managing the dual and simultaneous functions of information storage and processing. Although there is no direct evidence of a relation between central executive dysfunction and language comprehension difficulties in children with SLI, there are some data suggesting that these children have trouble flexibly allocating their resources to different aspects of language input during language learning tasks (Ellis Weismer & Hesketh, 1996; Johnston, Blatchley, & Olness, 1990) and to different linguistic operations during expressive language tasks (Dromi, Leonard, & Shteiman, 1993; Leonard, McGregor, & Allen, 1992). For example, it has been argued that these children may have trouble distributing their resources to both content words (specifically their serial order in sentences) and suffixes when learning language (Johnston et al., 1990) and to different mental operations (e.g., retrieving the linguistic property of a grammatical morpheme and at the same time retrieving and executing the motor program associated with the production of a morpheme) when talking (Leonard et al., 1992). More "direct" evidence of capacity limitations of the central executive has been reported by Oakhill et al. (1988) and Yuill et al. (1989) in school-age children who exhibit poor reading comprehension abilities.

The idea that some of the language performance difficulties (and variability) of children with SLI can be accounted for on the basis of their having greater trouble allocating and managing their resources also has been espoused by other researchers (e.g., Lahey & Bloom, 1994). With respect to comprehension, for example, Lahey and Bloom (1994) argue that successful comprehension is not a simple function or consequence of being able to manage the operations of WM alone. Rather, they propose that the efficiency with which a listener can allocate and manage his or her WM resources during language processing is a result of a complex interaction of child-internal factors and external/input factors, thereby making the relation between WM and language functioning reciprocal. Among these factors are (a) the ease with which a child can build and hold in WM the necessary mental representations, or "models," of the input (and, relatedly, the ability to automatically retrieve the language knowledge/processing procedures needed to construct the representations); (b) the content familiarity of the to-be-processed material; (c) the nature/structure of the to-be-processed material (e.g., decontextualized versus scripted/routine language); and (d) the presence/strength of contextual cues. Thus, sentence comprehension derives from a "synergistic interaction of several processes with each other, with context, and with the material to be processed" (p. 355).

A child with SLI, then, who is faced with having to simultaneously attend to multiple features (e.g., unfamiliar lexical items, multiple grammatical morphemes, complex and not well-learned syntactic structures) of a string of decontextualized utterances relating to an unfamiliar topic will undoubtedly have difficulty fully understanding what is said. This is because the many features in each incoming sentence will compete for and receive variable and even insufficient amounts of the child's limited WM resources. Moreover, because a certain amount of resources will have been allocated to storing what has already been fully or partially processed, even fewer resources will be available for processing new information. By contrast, the comprehension and retention of verbal material can be greatly facilitated if the input is familiar, predictable, and highly structured, and if the child can easily construct a mental representation of the input, as may be the case when he or she is listening to a story. Thus, the relation between memory functioning and language processing is by no means unidirectional (i.e., WM always facilitating comprehension).

CLINICAL IMPLICATIONS

Assessment suggestions

Central to the assessment process is determining to what extent a client's poor comprehension performance is related to deficiencies in linguistic knowledge versus difficulties managing his or her WM resources or to a combination of factors. Accordingly, one of the first steps of assessment is to try to determine the range and level of linguistic knowledge of the client. Then, given the considerable research evidence of a strong association between WM and comprehension, it would seem appropriate to obtain an estimate of the client's WM abilities. Unfortunately, however, there is little agreement on how best to assess WM. Furthermore, there are few standardized measures designed to assess WM. Despite these shortcomings, it is possible to assess clients' WM abilities and to make some reasonable inferences about how their sentence comprehension abilities are influenced by their ability to manage their WM resources. Such an assessment can be accomplished with the use of some conventional measures of memory, carefully constructed informal assessment protocols (motivated by the literature), and systematic task analyses and authentic language assessments. However, given the paucity of assessment instruments and lack of agreement on how best to measure WM, it is important that the reader understands that many of the following assessment techniques are offered as suggestions.

For young, preschool children the phonological loop component of WM can be reliably assessed using a variety of conventional memory measures, including standardized digit span and word span tasks, and through the use of informal nonsense word repetition tasks (Gathercole & Adams, 1993). Because all of these measures have been found to be significantly correlated with one another in this age group, Gathercole and Adams (1993) argue that conventional digit span and word span tasks are as sensitive to phonological loop functioning in young children as nonsense word repetition tasks. The digits forward tasks from the Weschler Intelligence Scale for Children-III (WISC-III; Wechsler, 1991) and the Test of Memory and Learning (Reynolds & Bigler, 1994) have the child recall a series of digits in the order they have been presented. The digits backward task from the WISC-III requires the child to repeat number series in reverse order. On the surface, this task would appear to be sensitive to the central executive component of WM because of its storage and processing requirements and not just to the storage buffer of the phonological loop. Those children who perform below age-level expectations on these tasks would be considered to have reduced phonological memory capacity.

Performance on measures of word span such as the Word Order subtest of the Kaufman Assessment Battery for Children (Kaufman & Kaufman, 1983) also can assess the capacity of the phonological loop in preschoolers. In this task, the child is presented lists of semantically unrelated words. With each new list, the number of to-be-recalled words increases by one. After each list the child is asked to recall the words in serial order. Again, a child who performs below age expectations would be considered to demonstrate reduced phonological memory capacity.

The nonsense word repetition task, in particular, has proved to be an especially sensitive index of phonological memory functioning in preschool and early school-age children. Whereas performance on digit span and word span tasks potentially could be mediated through the use of various mnemonic strategies (depending on the sophistication of the child), the repetition of nonsense words presumably requires greater reliance on phonological memory because the input is unknown and hence not subject to lexical influences. In this task, children are asked to repeat singly presented nonsense words varying in length from one to four or five syllables. A reduced phonological WM capacity would be indicated by a length effect—that is, markedly poorer repetition of three-, four-, and five-syllable items than one- and two-syllable items. In the absence of any normative data, the performance of the child with SLI should be compared with the performance of achieving children without SLI of similar age who demonstrate no difficulty on the same task. Although the repetition of nonsense words is influenced less by stimulus familiarity than digits and real words, SLPs still need to exercise care when constructing nonsense words so that the items do not closely resemble real words in phonological or syllabic structure (Dollaghan, Biber, & Campbell, 1993, 1995; Gathercole, Willis, Emslie, & Baddeley, 1991). This safeguard should ensure the creation of a task that is maximally sensitive to the operations of phonological WM.

For children who are school age and older, the central executive component of WM can be assessed through the use of a variety of creative, literature-driven, clinician-developed assessment procedures. When assessing the central executive, SLPs will need to focus on how well the client can simultaneously remember already-processed information while also processing new, incoming verbal information. A task that seems to fit the bill on each of these accounts is the Competing Language Processing Task (Gaulin & Campbell, 1994). In this task, the client is read simple sentences (e.g., "Trees have *leaves*," "Babies drive *trucks*," "Dishes can *whistle*"). Groups of sentences are presented in increasing set size, beginning with two sentences and ending with six. The client is asked to perform two mental activities. First, he or she is asked to respond to the truth value of each sentence by answering either true (yes) or false (no). Second, he or she is asked to remember the last word of each sentence, but in no particular order. Immediately following the last sentence of the set, he or she is asked to recall as many sentence-final words as he or she can. For the sentences above, the client would respond true, false, and false. After the third sentence, the client would then try to recall the words *leaves, trucks,* and *whistle*. The word recall element of the task provides an estimate of the client's WM capacity, in addition to an indication of how efficient the client is in allocating his or her limited WM resources. The processing component of WM is assessed by the client having to interpret the meaning of each sentence. Because Gaulin and Campbell provide preliminary normative data for children between the ages of 6 and 12, reasonable judgments about a client's WM capacity and ability to manage the dual functions of WM can be made, independent of complex language processing demands (e.g., listening to a lecture and taking notes).

A second type of task, one that is modeled after Oakhill et al. (1988) and one that is more proximal to everyday comprehension, is to read a client a story in which a potentially anomalous piece of information is presented and it needs to be resolved by integrating another piece of information with it. The key here is that the resolving information can systematically occur in a sentence before the anomalous sentence or following one or more intervening sentences. Clients with a limited central executive should be able to answer the probe question about why the anomaly occurred when the resolving information appears in the sentence immediately before or after the anomalous sentence, but not after several intervening sentences (Oakhill et al., 1988). Such a response pattern would suggest that the client has trouble storing previously comprehended information while simultaneously processing new information.

So far this chapter has dealt exclusively with tasks designed to assess the two components of WM, independent of complex language processing demands. The intent of these tasks is to try to establish some sort of baseline estimate of the client's WM abilities, with the assumption that if a child demonstrates poor WM functioning under these stripped down conditions, he or she in all likelihood also will show difficulties managing his or her WM resources during more taxing language processing activities. To derive more "ecologically valid" estimates of a client's WM functioning, the SLP will need to conduct careful task analyses (e.g., Lahey & Bloom, 1994) and authentic assessments of language functioning (e.g., Wiig, 1995). Both methods allow the SLP to examine the reciprocal relation between memory and language.

The purpose of a task analysis, for example, is to determine which aspect(s) of a variety of language processing tasks influences the efficiency with which the client can manage his or her WM resources. For instance, a student's WM resources may be exceeded when he or she is trying to process new lecture material containing new concepts and vocabulary and complex sentence structures presented in the absence of supporting contextual cues. The student also might demonstrate poor processing of a new genre of text (e.g., expository text) because its structure and organization are unfamiliar, despite the fact that the language content is well within his or her grasp. The same client, however, may have no difficulty managing the WM demands of a task in which he or she is asked to process familiar material or material that has a known inherent structure (e.g., narrative). Thus, task analyses by design allow the SLP to examine how a client's use of WM resources is influenced by the various child-internal and external/input factors discussed by Lahey and Bloom (1994). In short, to obtain as complete an estimate of a client's ability to manage his or her WM resources during input processing, the assessment process must, at a minimum, include tasks that systematically vary the cognitive load on comprehension (Lahey & Bloom, 1994).

Intervention suggestions

In light of the strong association between poor WM abilities and (a) reduced vocabulary growth in young children, (b) reading comprehension deficits in young and older individuals with reading impairments, and (c) compromised sentence comprehension in children with SLI, interventions designed to promote more efficient use of WM may prove beneficial to some children with SLI (Gathercole & Baddeley, 1993). Also, in the absence of any intervention data demonstrating that WM-based intervention approaches are contraindicated, it seems reasonable to offer such approaches to some children with SLI, with the intent to help them improve their sentence processing abilities. At the same time, however, we do not advocate an exclusively "specific skills"- or "process"-based approach to remediating all language comprehension problems of all children with SLI. Given the interrelatedness of memory and language functioning, WM-based interventions that disregard this reciprocal relationship will in all likelihood fall short in maximally facilitating the overall language processing abilities of the client. Below, several techniques are suggested for enhancing the WM abilities of children with SLI. Importantly, however, given the absence of any efficacy data, the reader needs to keep in mind that the following techniques are offered only as suggestions.

For those preschool children demonstrating poor phonological memory, Mann (1984) has suggested that naming letters and objects, remembering spoken sentences, and listening to stories and nursery rhymes might prove beneficial in promoting phonological memory abilities. Having children listen to and repeat nursery rhymes, in particular, would seem to be an especially useful activity because rhymes highlight the phonological structure of language (see Fazio, Chapter 4). Exposure to nursery rhymes gives young children the opportunity to attend to and discover the internal phonological structure of words. Another way of promoting phonological memory skills in preschool children may be to provide them with plenty of practice in repeating unfamiliar words or nonsense ("funny") words. Providing them with opportunities to perceive and repeat nonsense words in a game-like situation may facilitate their ability to abstract the combinatorial properties of novel phonological strings, which may in itself improve their abilities to represent input phonologically in WM. Relatedly, more active rhyming games could be played by an adult and a child. For instance, an adult and a child might play rhyming word games in which they take turns producing rhyming words. A stimulus word such as *sock* might be given by the adult and the child produces as many real words or nonwords as he or she can. The adult and child could also play what might be called a "gating game" in which the adult tells the child that he or she (adult) is thinking of a word and it begins, for example, with the sound /k/. The child is asked to guess the word that the adult is thinking of. After each guess by the child, the adult provides another sound (e.g., /kae:/). The adult provides as many phonemes as necessary until the child guesses the word. The purpose of the game is to enhance the child's appreciation of the phonological structure of words and the notion that words comprise discrete/isolable phonetic segments and the ability to store in WM the sounds that he or she hears. An additional benefit of these games is that they might foster metaphonological awareness in the child, given that he or she presumably "attends" to the phonological structure of the input during these activities.

Older, school-age children and adolescents with SLI who appear to demonstrate inefficient use of WM resources during sentence processing may benefit from acquiring a variety of strategies designed to enhance the functional capacity of their WM system. It is assumed that the following strategies would be especially appropriate for those individuals who do not demonstrate receptive language knowledge deficits. For these individuals, such strategies might serve to reduce the size of the input into more manageable processing units. However, for those individuals with language deficiencies, some of these strategies may not be as effective in enhancing comprehension. On the one hand, these strategies may provide just the right means to help these individuals retain the input for longer periods while they discover and learn the form/meaning of the sentences. On the other hand, for other individuals, it might be necessary to design a combination intervention in which specific language knowledge and memory strategies are taught. The one theme common to any approach that might be used is to try to help the client better understand his or her memory and language processing abilities, with the intent to provide greater motivation for his or her learning and using various strategies to facilitate verbal comprehension and retention.

One technique that can be taught is verbal rehearsal. If the individual does not already spontaneously use verbal rehearsal, he or she may need to be taught why, when, and how to use it. Although verbal rehearsal is a general STM-enhancing technique, it also is a technique that directly relates to the operation of WM. Recall that the phonological loop of WM comprises a verbal rehearsal component. Helping clients to spontaneously use rehearsal should better enable them to refresh and retain speech material that gains access to the phonological store. Relatedly, the client also may benefit from learning the more general STM-enhancing technique of chunking words contained in sentences into more manageable chunks. The client may benefit from learning how to create prosodic chunks corresponding to phrases or clauses, units that in turn could be more manageably rehearsed and refreshed. Such a strategy might provide the client a more efficient way of retaining speech input, thereby potentially facilitating his or her comprehension.

For speech material larger than the sentence, teaching individuals the technique of paraphrasing—which encompasses listening comprehension, organization, and verbal expression—may be especially useful for individuals in the elementary grades and beyond (Donahue & Pidek, 1993). The focus of paraphrasing would be to help the individual use his or her own words to condense a large amount of linguistic information into smaller, well-integrated units. By having individuals restate and rephrase material, comprehension, integration, and retention may be improved as a result of maximizing the operations of the central executive.

Although SLPs attempt to facilitate more efficient use of WM in their clients, they may at the same time also try to help their clients acquire more automatic and efficient linguistic retrieval abilities and language processing routines, thereby effectively increasing their WM capacity (Lahey & Bloom, 1994). For instance, activities that provide clients with directed practice at processing/interpreting various language forms (e.g., words, syntactic structures) that have been troublesome may promote more readily accessible language knowledge and more automatic language processing procedures. Relatedly, helping children learn the structure of larger, unfamiliar language forms (e.g., narratives, expository texts) also may promote more effective use of the client's WM. Many children with SLI may benefit from intervention that incorporates both WM-based and language-based goals and strategies.

•   •   •

Sentence understanding is a complex psycholinguistic event in which language-specific knowledge sources interact with various cognitive processes. This chapter explored the association between sentence comprehension and one of these cognitive processes, namely, WM in children with SLI. It was argued that the sentence comprehension problems of some children with SLI may be related to their difficulty managing their more limited WM resources. A model of WM developed by Baddeley and associates was offered as a framework within which SLPs can begin to examine the association between WM and sentence comprehension in their clients. However, because clients in "real-life" processing situations seldom behave exactly like subjects performing in controlled experiments, the reader should apply the Baddeley model (or some other model of WM) in principled ways to systematically examine how variations in processing load influence the sentence comprehension of their clients. Armed with knowledge about WM and its association with language processing, SLPs can continue to be as innovative as they always have been in assessing and treating the language learning and processing problems of children with SLI.

REFERENCES

Adams, A., & Gathercole, S. (1995). Phonological working memory and speech production in preschool children. *Journal of Speech and Hearing Research, 38*, 403–414.

Baddeley, A. (1986). Working memory and comprehension. In D. Broadbent, J. McGaugh, M. Kosslyn, N. Mackintosh, E. Tulving, & L. Weiskrantz (Eds.), *Working memory.* Oxford, England: Oxford University Press.

Baddeley, A., & Hitch, G. (1974). Working memory. In G. Bower (Ed.), *The psychology of learning and motivation* (Vol. 8, pp. 47–90). New York: Academic Press.

Baddeley, A., Vallar, G., & Wilson, B. (1987). Sentence comprehension and phonological memory: Some neuropsychological evidence. In M. Coltheart (Ed.), *Attention and performance XII: The psychology of reading* (pp. 507–529). Hove, England: Erlbaum.

Bar-Shalom, E., Crain, S., & Shankweiler, D. (1993). A comparison of comprehension and production abilities of good and poor readers. *Applied Psycholinguistics, 14*, 197–227.

Butterworth, B., Campbell, R., & Howard, D. (1986). The uses of short-term memory: A case study. *Quarterly Journal of Experimental Psychology, 38A*, 705–738.

Carpenter, P., Just, M., & Shell, P. (1990). What one intelligence test measures: A theoretical account of the processing in the Raven Progressive Matrices Test. *Psychological Review, 97*, 404–431.

Ceci, S., Ringstrom, M., & Lea, S. (1981). Do language learning disabled children have impaired memories? In search of underlying processes. *Journal of Learning Disabilities, 14*, 159–173.

Curtiss, S., & Tallal, P. (1991). On the nature of the impairment in language-impaired children. In J. Miller (Ed.), *Research on child language disorders: A decade of progress.* Austin, TX: PRO-ED.

Daneman, M., & Carpenter, P. (1983). Individual differences in integrating information between and within sentences. *Journal of Experimental Psychology: Learning, Memory, and Cognition, 9*, 561–584.

Dollaghan, C., Biber, M., & Campbell, T. (1993). Constituent syllable effects in a nonsense-word repetition task. *Journal of Speech and Hearing Research, 36*, 1051–1054.

Dollaghan, C., Biber, M., & Campbell, T. (1995). Lexical influences on nonword repetition. *Applied Psycholinguistics, 16*, 211–222.

Donahue, M., & Pidek, C. (1993). Listening comprehension and paraphrasing in content-area classrooms. *Journal of Childhood Communication Disorders, 15*, 35–42.

Dromi, E., Leonard, L., & Shteiman, M. (1993). The grammatical morphology of Hebrew-speaking children with specific language impairment: Some competing hypotheses. *Journal of Speech and Hearing Research, 36*, 760–771.

Ellis Weismer, S., & Hesketh, L. (1996). Lexical learning by children with specific language impairment: Effects of linguistic input presented at varying speaking rates. *Journal of Speech and Hearing Research, 39*, 177–190.

Engle, R., Cantor, J., & Carullo, J. (1992). Individual differences in working memory and comprehension: A test of four hypotheses. *Journal of Experimental Psychology: Learning, Memory, and Cognition, 18*, 972–992.

Gathercole, S., & Adams, A. (1993). Phonological working memory in very young children. *Developmental Psychology, 29*, 770–778.

Gathercole, S., & Baddeley, A. (1990a). Phonological memory deficits in language disordered children: Is there a causal connection? *Journal of Memory and Language, 29*, 336–360.

Gathercole, S., & Baddeley, A. (1990b). The role of phonological memory in vocabulary acquisition: A study of young children learning new words. *British Journal of Psychology, 81*, 439–454.

Gathercole, S., & Baddeley, A. (1993). *Working memory and language.* Hillsdale, NJ: Erlbaum.

Gathercole, S., Willis, C., Emslie, H., & Baddeley, A. (1991). The influences of number of syllables and wordlikeness on children's repetition of nonwords. *Applied Psycholinguistics, 12*, 349–367.

Gathercole, S., Willis, C., Emslie, H., & Baddeley, A. (1992). Phonological memory and vocabulary development during the early school years: A longitudinal study. *Developmental Psychology, 28*, 887–898.

Gaulin, C., & Campbell, T. (1994). Procedure for assessing verbal working memory in normal school-age children: Some preliminary data. *Perceptual and Motor Skills, 79*, 55–64.

Gillam, R., Cowan, N., & Day, L. (1995). Sequential memory in children with and without language impairment. *Journal of Speech and Hearing Research, 38*, 393–402.

Graham, N. (1980). Memory constraints in language deficiency. In F. Jones (Ed.), *Language disability in children* (pp. 69–84). Baltimore: University Press.

Graybeal, C. (1981). Memory for stories in language-impaired children. *Applied Psycholinguistics, 2*, 269–283.

James, D., van Steenbrugge, W., & Chiveralls, K. (1994). Underlying deficits in language-disordered children with central auditory processing difficulties. *Applied Psycholinguistics, 15,* 311–328.

Johnston, J., Blatchley, M., & Olness, G. (1990). Miniature language system acquisition by children with different learning proficiencies. *Journal of Speech and Hearing Research, 33,* 335–342.

Just, M., & Carpenter, P. (1992). A capacity theory of comprehension: Individual differences in working memory. *Psychological Review, 99,* 122–149.

Kail, R., Hale, C., Leonard, L., & Nippold, M. (1984). Lexical storage and retrieval in language impaired children. *Applied Psycholinguistics, 5,* 37–49.

Kaufman, A., & Kaufman, N. (1983). *Kaufman Assessment Battery for Children.* Circle Pines, MN: American Guidance Services.

King, J., & Just, M. (1991). Individual differences in syntactic processing: The role of working memory. *Journal of Memory and Language, 30,* 580–602.

Kintsch, W., & Van Dijk, T. (1978). Toward a model of text comprehension and production. *Psychological Review, 85,* 363–394.

Kirchner, D., & Klatzky, R. (1985). Verbal rehearsal and memory in language disordered children. *Journal of Speech and Hearing Research, 28,* 556–564.

Lahey, M., & Bloom, L. (1994). Variability and language learning disabilities. In G. Wallach & K. Butler (Eds.), *Language learning disabilities in school-age children and adolescents* (pp. 354–372). New York: Macmillan.

Leonard, L., McGregor, K., & Allen, G. (1992). Grammatical morphology and speech perception in children with specific language impairment. *Journal of Speech and Hearing Research, 35,* 1076–1085.

Mann, V. (1984). Longitudinal prediction and prevention of early reading difficulty. *Annals of Dyslexia, 34,* 117–136.

Marslen-Wilson, W., & Tyler, L. (1980). The temporal structure of spoken language understanding. *Cognition, 8,* 1–71.

Marslen-Wilson, W., & Welsh, A. (1978). Processing interactions and lexical access during word recognition in continuous speech. *Cognitive Psychology, 10,* 29–63.

Martin, R. (1987). Articulatory and phonological deficits in short-term memory and their relation to syntactic processing. *Brain and Language, 32,* 159–192.

Montgomery, J. (1995a). Examination of phonological working memory in specifically language impaired children. *Applied Psycholinguistics, 16,* 355–378.

Montgomery, J. (1995b). Sentence comprehension in children with specific language impairment: The role of phonological working memory. *Journal of Speech and Hearing Research, 38,* 177–189.

Oakhill, J., Yuill, N., & Parkin, A. (1988). Memory and inference in skilled and less skilled comprehenders. In M.M. Gruneberg, P.E. Morris, & R.N. Sykes (Eds.), *Practical aspects of memory: Current research and issues* (Vol. 2, pp. 315–320). Chichester, England: Wiley.

Reynolds, C., & Bigler, E. (1994). *Test of memory and learning*. Austin, TX: PRO-ED.

Sininger, Y., Klatzky, R., & Kirchner, D. (1989). Memory scanning speed in language disordered children. *Journal of Speech and Hearing Research, 32,* 289–297.

Vallar, G., & Baddeley, A. (1984). Phonological short-term store, phonological processing and sentence comprehension: A neuropsychological case study. *Cognitive Neuropsychology, 1,* 121–141.

van der Lely, H., & Howard, D. (1993). Children with specific language impairment: Linguistic impairment or short-term memory deficit? *Journal of Speech and Hearing Research, 36,* 1193–1207.

Wechsler, D. (1991). *Wechsler Intelligence Scale for Children* (3rd ed.). San Antonio, TX: Psychological Corporation.

Wiig, E. (1995). Assessments of adolescent language. *Seminars in Speech and Language, 16,* 14–31.

Yuill, N., Oakhill, J., & Parkin, A. (1989). Working memory, comprehension ability and the resolution of text anomaly. *British Journal of Psychology, 80,* 351–361.

3

—

Capacity Limitations in Working Memory: The Impact on Lexical and Morphological Learning by Children with Language Impairment

Susan Ellis Weismer

Do children with language deficits have particular limitations in their capacity to process and store information? This is the question that has recently been explored by a number of investigators who have proposed capacity limitation accounts of language disorders (Bishop, 1992; Carpenter, Miyake, & Just, 1994; Gathercole & Baddeley, 1990a, 1993; Johnston, 1994; Johnston & Smith, 1989; Kirchner & Klatzky, 1985; Lahey & Bloom, 1994; Montgomery, 1995). The basis for these claims varies from reports of specific constraints in phonological working memory (Gathercole & Baddeley, 1993; Montgomery, Chapter 2) to claims based on performance on nonverbal reasoning tasks (Bishop, 1992; Johnston, 1994). One reason for appealing to information processing frameworks is to attempt to capture the range of difficulties exhibited by children with specific language impairment (SLI). In addition to deficits in language functioning, it has been shown that children with SLI demonstrate certain perceptual and cognitive limitations even though they perform within normal range on standardized measures of nonverbal cognition (see comprehensive reviews by Bishop, 1992; Ellis Weismer, 1993; Johnston, 1994; Tallal, 1988). As proposed by Bishop (1992), a hypothesis of limited processing capacity would suggest that the amount of material to be integrated

This work was supported by the National Institute on Deafness and Other Communication Disorders, NIH Grant #1R29DC01101.

Top Lang Disord 1996;17(1):33–44

and the time available for completing these operations will determine the success that children with language impairment experience, rather than the type of mental representation required by a given task (e.g., phonological representations versus visual images).

LIMITED CAPACITY MODELS

Limited capacity models of information processing have been proposed by various investigators including Baddeley (1986), Case (1985), Just and Carpenter (1992), and Kahneman (1973). Although the focus and details of these theoretical frameworks vary, the main thesis of these models is that the human information processing system has limited cognitive resources that can be allocated to different tasks. When task demands exceed the available resources, both storage and processing suffer. A typical example of limited resource capacity that is often given pertains to driving a car. When road conditions are good, it is possible to manage the various tasks involved in driving fairly automatically while listening to the radio and conversing with a friend. However, under more difficult driving conditions such as icy roads or limited visibility caused by fog, it becomes necessary to turn off the radio or suspend the conversation to conserve available resources to meet the increased driving demands.

Language as a limited capacity system

This notion of a limited capacity system has been incorporated within various accounts of language processing (Baddeley, 1986; Bloom, 1993; Bock, 1982; Just & Carpenter, 1992). According to these views, success in comprehending and producing language relies on the ability to actively maintain and integrate linguistic information within working memory. Trade-offs are thought to occur within and across language domains as demands reach the limits of resources. Empirical support for these claims comes from investigations that have indicated an association between phonological working memory and vocabulary growth in developing children without language disorders (Gathercole & Baddeley, 1990b; Gathercole, Willis, Emslie, & Baddeley, 1992) and between working memory capacity and comprehension of syntactically complex sentences by adults (Carpenter et al., 1994; King & Just, 1991).

Within Baddeley's (1986) model, working memory consists of a supervisory component referred to as the *central executive,* along with modality-specific storage buffers including the visuospatial sketchpad and the articulatory loop system. With respect to processing verbal information, Baddeley's framework focuses on the role of the articulatory loop (a speech-based storage and rehearsal buffer). Just and Carpenter's (1992) view of working memory for language corresponds to the part of the central executive that handles verbal information and does not entail modality-specific buffers. According to their theory, language processing is constrained by individual differences in cognitive capacity, defined in terms of the maximum amount of activation available in working memory to support storage and processing. That is, Just and Carpenter contend that capacity limitations constrain language performance more in some people than others. Similarly, Lahey and Bloom (1994) discuss language and cognitive variation among and within children in terms of the limited capacity processor notion, drawing on the broader construct of mental models rather than focusing strictly on language. Lahey and Bloom use the term *mental models* (somewhat differently than used by Johnson-Laird, 1983) to refer to representations constructed and held in consciousness that include images and/or propositions of some type. Within this framework, one could account for difficulties that children with SLI demonstrate in linguistic processing as well as limitations on certain nonverbal tasks by proposing that these children are restricted in their ability to hold in mind and manipulate multiple pieces of information, especially when that information requires rapid sequential processing (Bishop, 1992; Ellis Weismer, 1993).

EVIDENCE FOR CAPACITY LIMITATIONS IN DISORDERED LANGUAGE

Claims that capacity limitations are implicated in language disorders are based on several lines of investigation, including indirect evidence suggesting trade-offs among selected language domains (such that increases in syntactic complexity, for example, are associated with decreases in semantic or phonological complexity and/or accuracy). Such linguistic trade-offs have been reported for both typically developing children without language disorders and those with various types of language disorders (Bloom, Lightbown, & Hood, 1975; Camarata & Schwartz, 1985; Masterson & Kamhi, 1992; Panagos & Prelock, 1982); however, Masterson and Kamhi (1992) failed to find differential patterns of trade-offs for normal language (NL) children and those with language learning disabilities. Capacity limitations also have been inferred from the types of restrictions that children with SLI have displayed on certain nonverbal reasoning tasks (e.g., Johnston & Smith, 1989; Kamhi, Nelson, Lee, & Gholson, 1985), although working memory has not been the focus of these studies.

Several investigations have involved more direct examination of verbal working memory abilities in children with SLI, focusing on phonological working memory capacity as conceptualized within Baddeley's model. Gathercole and Baddeley (1990a) found that children with SLI were significantly poorer than NL children matched on mental age or language level at recalling multisyllabic nonsense words on a repetition task. Based on these findings, they suggested that children with SLI have a reduced capacity to store phonological information. A subsequent study by van der Lely and Howard (1993), however, failed to replicate these findings (see exchange among Gathercole & Baddeley, 1995, and Howard & van der Lely, 1995, and Cowan, Chapter 1, regarding possible reasons for the conflicting results). In a recent investigation, Montgomery (1995) confirmed the original findings of Gathercole and Baddeley (1990a) using a nonword repetition task and further demonstrated a relation between phonological working memory and sentence comprehension in children with SLI. In the investigations described below, there has been an attempt to extend the exploration of capacity limitations in SLI to language *learning* as well as processing. The focus of these studies is on the role that rate factors play in capacity limitations, using Just and Carpenter's (1992) framework of working memory for language.

THE ROLE OF PROCESSING RATE IN CAPACITY LIMITATIONS

In many current theoretical frameworks, capacity is viewed in terms of function, rather than structure, such that it translates into work accomplished within a set time interval (Johnston, 1994). Thus, increases in the rate, efficiency, or automatization of processing can free resources in working memory with resulting increases in capacity; conversely, reduced rates and efficiency of processing can lead to capacity constraints (Case,

1985; Chi & Gallagher, 1982; Lahey & Bloom, 1994). Numerous investigations by Tallal and colleagues have demonstrated temporal processing deficits in children with SLI across tasks using verbal and nonverbal stimuli (Fellbaum, Miller, Tallal, & Curtiss, 1994; Johnston, Stark, Mellits, & Tallal, 1981; Tallal & Piercy, 1973; Tallal, Stark, & Mellits, 1985). Findings from these studies indicate that the amount of time required for sensory information processing by children with SLI is significantly greater than that required by NL children (Tallal, 1988). Furthermore, children with SLI whose performance was interpreted as being indicative of limited resource capacity have been reported to have reduced scanning speed on verbal memory tasks (Kirchner & Klatzky, 1985; Sininger, Klatzky, & Kirchner, 1989). It appears, therefore, that reduced rate of processing may be a factor in the purported capacity limitations in working memory for children with SLI.

Given the hypothesized relation between rate of processing and resource capacity, it can be argued that manipulations in presentation rates of incoming stimuli should influence the ability to process and store information. Various investigations have examined the effect of manipulating speaking rate on linguistic processing by individuals with different types of language disorders. Difficulties in processing language presented at fast speaking rates have been reported for children with auditory perceptual problems (Manning, Johnston, & Beasley, 1977) and those with learning disabilities (McNutt & Chi-Yen Li, 1980). Evidence of beneficial effects of reduced speaking rates on auditory comprehension has been reported for adults with aphasia (Lasky, Weidner, & Johnson, 1976; Pashek & Brookshire, 1982; Weidner & Lasky, 1976; but see Blumstein, Katz, Goodglass, Shrier, & Dworetsky, 1985), children with learning disabilities (McCroskey & Thompson, 1973), and children with acquired aphasia (Campbell & McNeil, 1985). Using a dual-processing paradigm in which primary and secondary sentences were presented simultaneously, Campbell and McNeil (1985) found that slowing the rate of the primary sentence resulted in improved comprehension of a secondary sentence presented at normal rate. They interpreted these findings within a limited capacity model, suggesting that the slower rate of presentation of the primary sentences freed cognitive resources that could then be allocated to the processing of the secondary sentences.

INVESTIGATIONS OF LEXICAL AND MORPHOLOGICAL LEARNING: IMPACT OF CAPACITY LIMITATIONS

The author and colleagues have been conducting a series of investigations exploring the influence of variations in presentation rate during lexical and morphological learning on working memory capacity in children with SLI (Ellis Weismer, 1994; Ellis Weismer & Hesketh, 1993, 1996). These investigators hypothesized that presentation of language models at fast speaking rates may exceed children's capacity limitations and lead to reduced learning of novel words and morphemes, whereas the additional processing time afforded by slow speaking rates may facilitate linguistic computation and storage, resulting in better learning. In addition, the investigators expected rate variations to have the greatest impact on language learning by children with SLI given their presumed restrictions in working memory capacity. A summary of the findings from the lexical studies is provided below, along with a discussion of preliminary results from an ongoing investigation of morphological learning based on a subset of 16 children (eight with SLI/eight NL) of the 40 children participating in the study for whom complete data are available.

Experimental tasks

In each of the investigations the same basic paradigm was used in which either novel vocabulary or morphological markers were trained. The rationale for using novel target forms, rather than real language targets, was to ensure equivalent levels of knowledge of the targets before training (this way none of the children had ever been exposed to the forms being trained). Children were shown a toy figure identified as Sam the Outerspace Man and told that they would learn some "funny-sounding" words in Sam's outerspace language to refer to his toys. Modeling procedures were used during one or two training sessions such that the novel target forms were repeatedly paired with a particular unusual object (designated as one of Sam's toys). During lexical training, sentences such as "Sam is by the kub" were spoken as Sam was placed next to the target object in a row of three unfamiliar objects. The three novel words being taught were consistently modeled at a certain speaking rate, either slow (2.8 syll/sec), normal (4.4 syll/sec), or fast (5.9 syll/sec) rate. Training sentences were prerecorded to carefully control the rate of presentation of the models. Thus, the different novel words were trained at various speaking rates so that a given child might always hear the sentences modeling /kub/ presented at fast rate, /pon/ presented at normal rate, and /ted/ presented at slow rate. Novel words consisted of either consonant-vowel-consonant forms (e.g., /pon/) or consonant-vowel-consonant-consonant forms (e.g., /bImp/). Following exposure trials in which the novel forms were modeled, children were asked to produce, comprehend, or recognize the targets.

The novel morpheme learning task was similar to the lexical task in that different morphemes were trained at varying speaking rates. Three distinct morphemes were trained to correspond with the meanings *part of, broken,* or *little one,* with each morpheme consistently presented at a particular rate. Children were taught to attach the morphemes to the end of real words (e.g., /boto/ to refer to a broken boat) and to novel words referring to unusual objects (e.g., /kub/ to refer to part of a kub). In addition to asking children to demonstrate comprehension and production of the training targets, the investigators included generalization items that required children to attach the novel morpheme to a different word than the one modeled in training.

Participants

Participants in these investigations were school-age children in kindergarten through third grade who were monolingual English speakers. All children demonstrated normal-range nonverbal cognitive abilities and normal hearing at the time of testing. The children with SLI had previously been diagnosed and were receiving speech-language services in their schools for a language disorder. They exhibited language abilities that were below age-level expectations based on various standardized tests and on language sample analyses. Approximately half of the children with SLI exhibited only expressive language delays, whereas the others had both receptive and expressive deficits. The NL children had no history of delayed development in any area and performed within age-level expectations on measures of language comprehension and production.

Lexical learning results

The initial investigation of lexical learning (Ellis Weismer & Hesketh, 1993) indicated that variations in the speaking rate at which models were presented significantly influenced the ability of kindergartners to comprehend and produce novel vocabulary. Both the group with SLI and the NL group showed better understanding of novel words that had been trained at slow rate than at fast rate. Furthermore, children correctly produced significantly more novel words trained at normal rate than fast rate and significantly more words trained at slow compared with fast rate. Although these effects were found for both groups in this limited sample of children, there was a clear trend for the children with SLI to display greater responsiveness to rate variations than the NL children.

A follow-up investigation of novel word learning was conducted with somewhat older school-age children (mean age of 7 years) (Ellis Weismer, 1994; Ellis Weismer & Hesketh, 1996). Rate effects were most apparent on the production of novel words, rather than influencing children's ability to comprehend or recognize words. The school-age children in that study evidenced relatively high levels of performance on the comprehension and recognition items, but had more difficulty with the production items. Therefore, it follows that the impact of variations in presentation rate would be most obvious on the items that maximally stretched children's ability to process and store information in working memory (i.e., production of novel words). Findings indicated that children with SLI produced significantly fewer novel words correctly that had been trained at fast rate than normal rate. Furthermore, the children with SLI demonstrated significantly poorer production of words trained at fast rate than NL children matched on mental age or vocabulary level. Thus, rapid presentation rates had a much greater impact on word learning for children with SLI than for their NL peers. These findings imply a special restriction in processing capacity within working memory for the children with SLI.

An attempt was made to determine the nature of the difficulty that children with SLI had in producing novel words trained at fast rate. In particular, the investigators were interested in whether these children's poor performance was related to phonological working memory constraints or more generalized capacity constraints. An error analysis of children's production of the fast rate targets provided evidence for the impact of capacity limitations on phonological storage. That is, children with SLI exhibited significantly more errors that involved substitutions of real words for novel words, changes in syllable shape, and vowel errors than the NL children. It also was the case, however, that children with SLI mislabeled objects significantly more often than NL children. That is, they would recall the phonological form of a novel word, but would match up the wrong word and toy. Errors of this type implicate additional difficulties with association processes involved in mapping labels to appropriate referents, instead of pointing solely to a deficit in phonological memory. These findings are consistent with Just and Carpenter's framework, which suggests that capacity limitations might affect various aspects of lexical processing and storage and would not be restricted to problems in storing phonological information.

Contrary to previous investigations that have reported beneficial effects of slowed rate on auditory comprehension for adults with aphasia (e.g., Pashek & Brookshire, 1982), presentation of target forms at slow rate did not result in significantly better performance for children with SLI as a group. The author has speculated elsewhere (Ellis Weismer & Hesketh, 1993, 1996) that task differences may have played a role in these discrepant findings. That is, prior studies have used paragraphs or longer sentences, whereas this task consisted of embedding target words within relatively short (five-syllable) sentences. It may be the case that the distinction between linguistic input presented at normal versus slow rates would be more apparent at the connected discourse level because of cumulative effects of increased processing time and reduced processing load. Even though significant group differences were not observed, individual analyses were revealing from a clinical perspective. For example, examination of individual children's patterns of performance across the three rate conditions in the second lexical learning study (Ellis Weismer & Hesketh, 1993, 1996) indicated that 6 of 16 (38%) of the children with SLI (but none of the NL children) demonstrated consistent benefits of slow rate presentation with respect to comprehension scores. Eight of the 16 children with SLI (50%) evidenced improved production abilities under the slow rate condition, as did a few of the younger NL children.

Morphological learning results

Morpheme learning task

Preliminary results indicated that, as expected, children with SLI demonstrated significantly poorer overall learning of novel morphemes than their NL peers. The performance of the NL children was not significantly affected by rate variations. That is, their scores on the morpheme learning task were roughly equivalent under the three rate conditions. However, the group with SLI demonstrated significantly poorer production of items trained at fast rate than those trained at normal rate (37% compared with 67% accuracy). As was the case for the lexical learning task, slow rate did not lead to improved performance for the SLI group as a whole on these short stimulus sentences.

Dual-processing task

In addition to the morpheme learning task, all children received two tasks designed to assess aspects of working memory for verbal material. One task was a dual-processing task in which children were asked to respond to two tape-recorded instructions presented simultaneously (one spoken by a man and the other by a woman). For example, the child would hear the woman say "Pick up the white square and the blue square" as the man was saying "Put the little star on the big house." The effect is similar to situations in which someone asks you a question while you are listening to the news on TV. Children were instructed to try to remember what the woman had said and do that first, and then to do what the man had told them. This task was an adaptation of the dual-processing paradigm used by Campbell and McNeil (1985), in which two auditory comprehension measures were presented under competing (i.e., dual-processing) and noncompeting listening conditions. All children were expected to perform more poorly under the difficult competing listening condition than on the noncompeting condition when sentences were presented individually. The question of interest was whether the children with SLI would have *relatively* more difficulty with dual processing than the NL children. The differences in the groups' comprehension scores on the noncompeting compared with competing conditions for sentences spoken at normal rate indicated that the group with SLI exhibited disproportionate decrements in dual processing in comparison with the NL group. That is, the difference between the comprehension scores for the noncompeting condition (when sentences were presented individually) and the competing condition (when those same sentences were presented together) was significantly greater for the children with SLI than those with NL. These preliminary findings suggest that children with SLI may have restrictions in working memory capacity that make it extremely difficult to maintain multiple pieces of linguistic information at the same time.

Verbal working memory task

A second task that was used was a measure developed by Gaulin and Campbell (1994) to assess verbal working memory in school-age children. Their measure, the Competing Language Processing Task, was based on a listening span task by Daneman and Carpenter (1980) designed to evaluate adults' verbal memory span. In the version developed for children, groups of two to six short sentences are presented and children must demonstrate comprehension by responding true or false to each sentence. In addition, they are asked to recall the last word of each sentence after all of the sentences in a group have been presented. The comprehension aspect of the task is easy, consisting of simple sentences such as "Pumpkins are purple." Preliminary findings revealed that both groups of children exhibited similar, high levels of performance (more than 95% accuracy) on the true/false comprehension items. However, the children with SLI demonstrated significantly poorer word recall performance (ability to recall the last word in each sentence for sets of sentences) than the NL children in this study. Furthermore, the mean score for the group with SLI fell two standard deviations below the mean for that age level based on the norms established by Gaulin and Campbell (1994). These tentative findings, such as those from the dual-processing task, suggest that children with SLI have limitations in verbal working memory capacity.

Relation between morpheme learning and memory

Preliminary analyses were conducted to assess the relation between children's performances on the two working memory measures and the morpheme learning task. A positive, moderate correlation was found between the ability of children with SLI to produce novel morphemes trained at fast rate and their word recall scores on the verbal memory span task. Similarly, their performance on the fast rate targets was moderately correlated with their performance on the dual-processing task. In other words, for the children with SLI, performance on these indices of working memory seems to be related to some extent to their performance on the most difficult items on the morpheme learning task—namely, those trained at fast rate. Of course, all of the findings from the investigation of morphological learning are preliminary and will need to be confirmed with the larger sample.

Conclusion

The results of the novel lexical learning investigations, as well as the tentative findings from the novel morpheme learning study, indicate that variations in the presentation rate of verbal information influence the performance of children with SLI. Preliminary findings from the measures assessing verbal working memory provide further support for the contention that capacity constraints play a role in language disorders. These results add to the prior findings regarding restrictions in verbal working memory exhibited by children with SLI (Gathercole & Baddeley, 1990a; Montgomery, 1995) and suggest that these limitations affect both processing and learning of new language forms.

Implications for intervention

These findings indicate that variations in the speaking rate at which linguistic models are presented affect children's ability to learn language, suggesting that clinicians should pay attention not only to the content of the models provided during intervention, but also to the manner in which they are presented. Children with SLI appear to have particular difficulty processing and storing verbal information presented at fast rates; therefore, fast speaking rates should be avoided in instructional situations. Although the group as a whole did not demonstrate better learning with slow presentation rates, individual analyses indicated that some children with SLI do benefit from models presented at slow rates. Using the same novel word learning paradigm used in the investigations of speaking rate variations, the researchers also found that children with SLI produced significantly more novel words correctly that had received emphatic stress during training compared with words that received no special emphasis (Ellis Weismer, Hesketh, Hollar, & Neylon, 1994). Apparently, the use of emphatic stress on the target word helped to direct the children's limited resources to the new information to be learned, improving their ability to later recall the novel words. Although experimental group findings can serve as a general guide for determining appropriate teaching procedures, it is important to anticipate considerable variability in children's responses to variations in linguistic input such as these and to recognize the need for individual trial teaching to assess the effect of these modifications on a particular child's language learning.

Now consider the broader treatment implications of findings that suggest that children with SLI have capacity limitations. To begin, interventionists should analyze the demands placed on working memory by a specific task and attempt to reduce processing loads when first introducing new language forms. Thus, by ensuring that other aspects of the task require minimal cognitive resources, a greater proportion of available resources can be dedicated to the processing and storage of the new information. For example, when teaching new vocabulary, start with words containing sounds that the child can easily produce rather than more complex phonetic forms. When targeting new syntactic structures, use highly familiar vocabulary so that the child can focus primarily on the grammatical aspect of the sentence. Lahey and Bloom (1994) made similar recommendations with respect to intervention for older children with language learning disabilities. They suggested, for example, that initial attempts in teaching narrative construction might focus on mental models that are easily constructed, using simple syntactic constructions and familiar vocabulary, and deal with material that is affectively neutral rather than emotionally charged. As treatment progresses, these variables can be adjusted so that the child has the opportunity to produce narratives under increasingly difficult conditions.

Clinicians also can seek to establish teaching contexts that can facilitate the child's ability to access event knowledge from long-term memory, thereby reducing the processing load in working memory. This is one of the basic assumptions underlying the use of script-based language intervention approaches (Constable, 1986; Kim & Lombardino, 1991). In other words, when new language forms are introduced within the context of a familiar routine (such as snack time in a preschool classroom), the child has clear expectations about the sequence of events, the roles various people assume, and so forth. Presumably, scripted events allow the child to focus fewer cognitive resources on the activity per se, with additional resources then being available for language learning.

Finally, clinicians can mitigate capacity limitations in children with SLI by working to increase automaticity of newly acquired language skills. As more aspects of linguistic processing become automatic, fewer resources are used so that the net effect is increased capacity. Automaticity is accomplished through practice. To return to the earlier example of driving a car, it is only through considerable practice that certain components of the driving task become automatized, freeing resources for other concurrent activities under typical driving conditions. As noted by Lahey and Bloom (1994), practice does not necessarily mean engaging in drill-type activities. Instead, clinicians can promote automaticity by providing repeated opportunities for meaningful use of particular language forms and functions and by firmly establishing language skills before advancing to new goals. By accommodating potential processing capacity limitations in these ways, clinicians may promote better language learning in children with language deficits.

REFERENCES

Baddeley, A. (1986). *Working memory.* Oxford, England: Clarendon Press.

Bishop, D. (1992). The underlying nature of specific language impairment. *Journal of Child Psychology and Psychiatry, 33,* 3–66.

Bloom, L. (1993). *The transition from infancy to language: Acquiring the power of expression.* Cambridge, England: Cambridge University Press.

Bloom, L., Lightbown, P., & Hood, L. (1975). Structure and variation in child language. *Monographs of the Society for Research on Child Development, 40*(2).

Blumstein, S., Katz, B., Goodglass, J., Shrier, R., & Dworetsky, B. (1985). The effects of slowed speech on auditory comprehension in aphasia. *Brain and Language, 24,* 246–265.

Bock, J.K. (1982). Toward a cognitive psychology of syntax: Information processing contributions to sentence formulation. *Psychological Review, 89,* 1–47.

Camarata, S., & Schwartz, R. (1985). Production of action words and object words: Evidence for a relationship between semantics and phonology. *Journal of Speech and Hearing Research, 28,* 323–330.

Campbell, T., & McNeil, M. (1985). Effects of presentation rate and divided attention on auditory comprehension in children with an acquired language disorder. *Journal of Speech and Hearing Research, 28,* 513–520.

Carpenter, P., Miyake, A., & Just, M. (1994). Working memory constraints in comprehension: Evidence from individual differences, aphasia, and aging. In M.A. Gersbacher (Ed.), *Handbook of psycholinguistics* (pp. 1075–1122). San Diego, CA: Academic Press.

Case, R. (1985). *Intellectual development: Birth to adulthood.* New York: Academic Press.

Chi, M., & Gallagher, J. (1982). Speed of processing: A developmental source of limitation. *Topics in Learning and Learning Disabilities, 2,* 23–32.

Constable, C. (1986). The application of scripts in the organization of language intervention contexts. In K. Nelson (Ed.), *Event knowledge: Structure and function in development* (pp. 205–230). Hillsdale, NJ: Lawrence Erlbaum.

Daneman, M., & Carpenter, P. (1980). Individual differences in working memory and reading. *Journal of Verbal Learning and Verbal Behavior, 19,* 450–466.

Ellis Weismer, S. (1993). Perceptual and cognitive deficits in children with specific language impairment: Implications for diagnosis and intervention. In H. Grimm & H. Skowronek (Eds.), *Language acquisition problems and reading disorders: Aspects of diagnosis and intervention* (pp. 75–101). Berlin, Germany: Walter de Gruyter.

Ellis Weismer, S. (1994). *Factors influencing novel word learning and linguistic processing in children with specific language impairment.* Invited talk at the 15th Annual Symposium on Research in Child Language Disorders, Madison, WI.

Ellis Weismer, S., & Hesketh, L. (1993). The influence of prosodic and gestural cues on novel word acquisition by children with specific language impairment. *Journal of Speech and Hearing Research, 36,* 1013–1025.

Ellis Weismer, S., & Hesketh, L. (1996). Lexical learning by children with specific language impairment: Effects of linguistic input presented at varying speaking rates. *Journal of Speech and Hearing Research, 39,* 177–190.

Ellis Weismer, S., Hesketh, L., Hollar, C., & Neylon, C. (1994). *The role of emphatic stress in lexical learning.* Poster presented at the annual convention of the American Speech-Language-Hearing Association, New Orleans, LA.

Fellbaum, C., Miller, S., Tallal, P., & Curtiss, S. (1994). *Evidence for the relation between temporal processing deficit and specific language impairment.* Paper presented at the 15th Annual Symposium on Research in Child Language Disorders, Madison, WI.

Gathercole, S., & Baddeley, A. (1990a). Phonological memory deficits in language disordered children: Is there a causal connection? *Journal of Memory and Language, 29,* 336–360.

Gathercole, S., & Baddeley, A. (1990b). The role of phonological memory in vocabulary acquisition: A study of young children learning new words. *British Journal of Psychology, 81,* 439–454.

Gathercole, S., & Baddeley, A. (1993). *Working memory and language processing.* Hove, East Sussex, England: Lawrence Erlbaum.

Gathercole, S., & Baddeley, A. (1995). Short-term memory may yet be deficient in children with language impairments: A comment on van der Lely & Howard (1993). *Journal of Speech and Hearing Research, 38,* 463–466.

Gathercole, S., Willis, C., Emslie, H., & Baddeley, A. (1992). Phonological memory and vocabulary development during the early school years: A longitudinal study. *Developmental Psychology, 28,* 887–898.

Gaulin, C., & Campbell, T. (1994). Procedure for assessing verbal working memory in normal school-age children: Some preliminary data. *Perceptual and Motor Skills, 79,* 55–64.

Howard, D., & van der Lely, H. (1995). Specific language impairment in children is *not* due to a short-term memory deficit: Response to Gathercole and Baddeley. *Journal of Speech and Hearing Research, 38,* 466–472.

Johnson-Laird, P. (1983). *Mental models.* Cambridge, MA: Harvard University Press.

Johnston, J. (1994). Cognitive abilities of children with language impairment. In R. Watkins & M. Rice (Eds.), *Specific language impairment in children* (pp. 107–121). Baltimore: Brookes.

Johnston, J., & Smith, L. (1989). Dimensional thinking in language impaired children. *Journal of Speech and Hearing Research, 32,* 33–38.

Johnston, R., Stark, R., Mellits, E., & Tallal, P. (1981). Neurological status of language-impaired and normal children. *Annals of Neurology, 10,* 159–163.

Just, M., & Carpenter, P. (1992). A capacity theory of comprehension: Individual differences in working memory. *Psychological Review, 99*, 122–149.

Kahneman, D. (1973). *Attention and effort.* Englewood Cliffs, NJ: Prentice Hall.

Kamhi, A., Nelson, L., Lee, R., & Gholson, B. (1985). The ability of language-disordered children to use and modify hypotheses in discrimination learning. *Applied Psycholinguistics, 6*, 435–451.

Kim, Y., & Lombardino, L. (1991). The efficacy of script context in language comprehension intervention with children who have mental retardation. *Journal of Speech and Hearing Research, 34*, 845–857.

King, J., & Just, M. (1991). Individual differences in syntactic processing: The role of working memory. *Journal of Memory and Language, 30*, 580–602.

Kirchner, D., & Klatzky, R. (1985). Verbal rehearsal and memory in language disordered children. *Journal of Speech and Hearing Research, 28*, 556–564.

Lahey, M., & Bloom, L. (1994). Variability and language learning disabilities. In G. Wallach & K. Butler (Eds.), *Language learning disabilities in school-age children and adolescents* (pp. 354–372). New York: Macmillan.

Lasky, E., Weidner, W., & Johnson, J. (1976). Influence of linguistic complexity, rate of presentation, and interphrase pause time on auditory-verbal comprehension of adult aphasic patients. *Brain and Language, 3*, 386–395.

Manning, W., Johnston, K., & Beasley, D. (1977). The performance of children with auditory perceptual disorders on a time-compressed speech discrimination measure. *Journal of Speech and Hearing Disorders, 42*, 77–84.

Masterson, J., & Kamhi, A. (1992). Linguistic trade-offs in school-age children with and without language disorders. *Journal of Speech and Hearing Research, 35*, 1064–1075.

McCroskey, R., & Thompson, N. (1973). Comprehension of rate controlled speech by children with specific learning disabilities. *Journal of Learning Disabilities, 6*, 621–628.

McNutt, J., & Chi-Yen Li, J. (1980). Repetition of time altered sentences by normal and learning disabled children. *Journal of Learning Disabilities, 13*, 25–29.

Montgomery, J. (1995). Sentence comprehension in children with specific language impairment: The role of phonological working memory. *Journal of Speech and Hearing Research, 38*, 177–189.

Panagos, J., & Prelock, P. (1982). Phonological constraints on the sentence productions of language-disordered children. *Journal of Speech and Hearing Research, 25*, 171–177.

Pashek, G., & Brookshire, R. (1982). Effects of rate of speech and linguistic stress on auditory paragraph comprehension of aphasic individuals. *Journal of Speech and Hearing Research, 25*, 377–383.

Sininger, Y., Klatzky, R., & Kirchner, D. (1989). Memory scanning speed in language disordered children. *Journal of Speech and Hearing Research, 32*, 289–297.

Tallal, P. (1988). Developmental language disorders. In J. Kavanagh & T. Truss, Jr. (Eds.), *Learning disability proceedings from the national conference* (pp. 181–272). Parkton, MD: York Press.

Tallal, P., & Piercy, M. (1973). Developmental aphasia: Impaired rate of non-verbal processing as a function of sensory modality. *Neuropsychologia, 11*, 389–398.

Tallal, P., Stark, R., & Mellits, D. (1985). Identification of language-impaired children on the basis of rapid perception and production skills. *Brain and Language, 25*, 314–322.

van der Lely, H., & Howard, D. (1993). Children with specific language impairment: Linguistic impairment or short-term memory deficit? *Journal of Speech and Hearing Research, 36*, 1193–1207.

Weidner, W., & Lasky, E. (1976). Interaction of rate and complexity of stimulus on the performance of adult aphasic subjects. *Brain and Language, 3*, 34–70.

4
—

Serial Memory in Children with Specific Language Impairment: Examining Specific Content Areas for Assessment and Intervention

Barbara B. Fazio

Certain cognitive tasks require recalling not only a set of items but also the precise sequence of items. For example, to count the number of cookies on a plate, one must remember all the appropriate number words *in a specified order*. Memory for item order (serial memory) requires a mechanism that permits remembering two types of information—the item itself and its location in the sequence. Different labels used to refer to this type of memory are *serial memory, sequential memory,* or *memory for item order.* These terms all refer to the verbatim recall of a sequence of material. For the sake of consistency, the term *serial memory* will be used throughout this chapter.

Serial memory is seen in myriad cognitive and linguistic tasks each day. For example, one is consciously aware of remembering the serial order of items when memorizing a new telephone number or when attempting to remember directions to a new acquaintance's house. Older children and adults have learned that repetition keeps information in conscious memory. Serial memory also is used to retrace one's steps to remember the last place keys were left, when the total price of two store items is calculated, or when a topic of conversation is recalled after a distraction. Similarly, young children's school days are filled with serial memory tasks such as saying the number words in an invariant order ("seven, eight, nine, TEN!"), or singing songs and reciting rhymes ("Hey, diddle, diddle, the cat and the fiddle"). Serial memory also plays a role in understanding teacher

Top Lang Disord 1996;17(1):58–71

directions ("Put your things away, come to the circle, and sit with your legs crossed").

Serial memory limitations clearly affect cognitive abilities of children with specific language impairment (SLI). SLI is used here to refer to a heterogeneous group of children who despite scoring within normal limits on tests of nonverbal reasoning abilities, display poor performance on language tasks (Lahey, 1988). Research into serial memory difficulties for children with SLI is still in its early stages. The focus of this chapter is confined to young children and to two specific domains (one that affects children's basic mathematical knowledge and one that may influence children's beginning reading abilities). Specific assessment and intervention recommendations that follow from current research are addressed rather than sweeping generalities about "children with sequencing problems."

SERIAL MEMORY AND LANGUAGE USE

Children and adults store and produce myriad rote phrases. These phrases appear to be stored as one unit (e.g., "didjaknow?"). The usefulness of such formulaic phrases is in their economy. Given that such phrases might be stored and retrieved as one unit, they are quickly retrieved from memory; hence, using formulaic phrases increases language processing speed and efficiency (Peters, 1983).

The literature on early language development includes several descriptions of formulaic expressions (or frozen forms) that are found in very young children's speech, such as "Give me dat" (e.g., Bates, Bretherton, & Snyder, 1988). Formulaic speech also plays a role in preschool children's vocabulary. There are numerous social control phrases such as "It's my turn," "I don't wanna," or "I have something to say" that are particularly useful when they are interacting with other children (Peters, 1983). Preschool children also learn memorized sequences of connected speech such as counting, nursery rhymes, and reciting the alphabet.

Although we see young language users producing formulaic speech, however, there has been little attention to rote mechanisms in language learning or use. Peters (1983) suggested that there appears to be a theoretical bias in child language research against viewing rote memorization as a useful strategy for language users. In part, this may be a reaction to behavioristic (stimulus–response) models of language learning. However, there is clear evidence that rote serial memory plays a critical role in several cognitive domains, and there are serious consequences when rote linguistic sequences are inadequately stored, retrieved, or both.

SERIAL MEMORY DEFICITS IN CHILDREN WITH SLI

Several studies suggest that children with SLI have particular difficulty on tasks requiring immediate, verbatim ordered recall. For example, children with SLI have been found to have difficulty in tests of auditory digit span, that is, the longest sequence of digits that can be repeated in a correct sequence after one presentation (Gathercole & Baddeley, 1990) and in recalling lists of words (Kirchner & Klatzky, 1985). The main requirement of these tasks is to maintain the order of the items.

Problems in maintaining the serial order of information (serial memory) in the performance of children with SLI are seen in reciting nursery rhymes (Fazio, in press). Children appear to learn nursery rhymes by rote. Given the unusual vocabulary and archaic phrase structure, it is likely that children memorize each line (Maclean, Bryant, & Bradley, 1987). Fazio (in press) found that children with SLI had problems remembering lines of common nursery rhymes and often recalled rhymes in an unconventional order. By the same token, children with SLI have difficulty with maintaining the correct sequence of number words on various counting tasks such as rote counting to 20.

What causes problems with serial memory?

Most current memory models describe serial memory as the consequence of working memory. Working memory is the process that allows for ongoing access of a small number of items of information in conscious awareness. To keep information available in memory, it must be repeated, that is, rehearsed or reorganized (categorized) or it quickly fades (see Cowan, Chapter 1). In language processing, working memory holds incoming linguistic material while the underlying meaning is found. The great usefulness of the notion of working memory is that it provides an explanation for how information is kept in mind long enough to make sense of sequences of words, to process information in and out of long-term storage, or to solve problems.

A critical aspect of many memory models involves processing capacity, that is, the total amount of cognitive resources available for use in a task

(Baddeley, 1986; Just & Carpenter, 1992). Conscious attentional resources are needed when learning new tasks. However, such attention produces a strain on the limited resources of working memory (Baddeley, 1986). Tasks that draw substantially from the limited pool of resources are termed *controlled tasks*. Tasks that do not require extensive resources are considered *automatic*. Tasks become automatic through extensive practice (Logan, 1988). For example, as anyone who has recently tried to arrange a filing system knows, adults have recited the alphabet thousands of times. This task has become automatic through practice. However, for the very young, this task demands many more resources. Over time, thousands of such tasks become overlearned so that adults are faster and more efficient information processors. Many theorists maintain that there is no substantial increase in overall working memory capacity as children mature to adulthood (e.g., Kail, 1990). Instead, they suggest that there is a functional increase of processing capacity as a result of greater automaticity.

A second important aspect of working memory relates to the predominance of phonological content. For example, in Baddeley's (1986) model of working memory, codes used to represent verbal material on tasks requiring immediate verbatim ordered recall are composed primarily of the phonological features of the stimuli. In other words, only the phonological form of the word is needed for immediate serial recall. (The semantic features of the words may not be necessary.) Difficulty with phonological coding should affect performance on any task requiring brief verbatim storage of verbal information. Therefore, one explanation for the source of the sequencing problems seen in children with SLI is poor phonological memory storage (Gathercole & Baddeley, 1990). The precise mechanisms that are the source of phonological storage problems are unknown, although Gathercole and Baddeley (1993) suggest that the capacity of the phonological store is reduced in children with SLI.

Phonological storage capacity is not the only viable explanation for serial memory problems in children with SLI. As discussed earlier, several researchers envision capacity not as a structure but as a function of processing efficiency (e.g., Kail, 1990). Instead of stemming from poor capacity for the storage of phonological information, serial memory problems may be the result of slow and inefficient processing (e.g., Kirchner & Klatzky, 1985). Children with SLI may not develop the ability to process phonological information as readily as children without SLI. This lack of ability would produce a generalized impairment in the efficiency with which children with SLI can process temporal information (e.g., Sininger, Klatzky, & Kirchner, 1989). As a result of this phonological inefficiency, the encoding of serial information may suffer. The encoding process (that is, how items are entered into memory) may be unreliable, inconsistent, and open to interference (Gillam, Cowan, & Day, 1995). This fits with the earlier discussion on viewing the information processing system as a limited capacity processor. When phonological processing stresses the system, temporal (serial) information may be easily lost.

Phonological or semantic storage and retrieval abilities also may affect the recall of rote linguistic sequences. For example, many children with SLI have word-finding problems (e.g., Kail & Leonard, 1986). Children with word-finding problems may substitute or repeat words or use nonspecific terms such as *thing* (German, 1992). They often display deficits in tests of single word retrieval or in tasks that require fast, accurate names for colors, numbers, or common objects (Denckla & Rudel, 1976; Fazio, 1996).

Problems with serial memory may compromise a child's ability to understand and produce language. They also impede children's acquisition of academic skills that demand a heavy memory load for sequences of linguistic material. The following discussion focuses on two specific domains: learning early mathematics and preliteracy rhyme knowledge. Three questions and their answers follow: What role does serial memory play in certain academic areas? How can serial memory problems be assessed in specific academic domains? What does current research suggest are strong contenders for effective intervention strategies?

SERIAL MEMORY AND THE DEVELOPMENT OF MATHEMATICS

Adults who effortlessly use the intricate system of English number terms may forget how difficult it must be to master. One of the most important elements of this system is using number terms for rote counting. In counting objects, the child needs to know all the names for number terms, and these number terms must be learned in the correct sequence. The child must somehow keep track of which ones have been counted (and which ones still need to be counted). Usually children point or touch each object to keep track of which ones to count (but they need to make sure they do not skip an object or touch the same object twice). Then, when each item has been "tagged" (e.g., touched only once), they need to know that the last number word they spoke represents the size of the group of objects.

From the example preceding, children demonstrate several abilities: the knowledge that there is an individual number word for each number concept, that number words must be recited in a given sequence, that there is a one-to-one correspondence between objects to be counted and number words, and that the last word spoken represents the total number of objects in a set. The ability to recite a set of sequenced number terms (i.e., rote counting) provides the basis for symbolically representing quantities (Fuson, 1988).

Fuson (1988) reviewed the literature on children without SLI and their development of number words and contended that number words are acquired in a sequence of steps. At first, children learn to recite the number words as if they were a chant or rhyme without any association to number concepts. These unanalyzed strings of sounds have the same phonology as other words, and they are conventional, but they are not yet symbolic. Next, number words are used to represent a nonspecific quantity, for instance, "I want three" referring to "I want some." Later, children learn that number words also are used in one-to-one correspondence to count objects. Counting an object twice or skipping an object will lead to the wrong answer. Learning to count actual objects helps to break the stream of number words into individual segments (Resnick, 1983). Counting pushes the child to reanalyze the number terms as a representation of exact quantity. Now when children ask for four cookies, they carefully count to make sure they did not get fleeced. Children observed at this point in number development reveal that they have learned that the last word spoken represents the total number of items contained in the set (Fuson, Pergament, & Lyons, 1985).

Past research has shown that having a consistent order of number words (i.e., a block of correctly sequenced number words) is a critical component to learning the number system (Fuson, 1988). The impact of knowing the correct sequence of number words lies in its effect on later mathematical learning. Rote counting appears to be the bootstrap that allows one admission into the domain of numbers (Carpenter & Moser, 1984). Not knowing the language associated with counting is therefore a stumbling block; it impedes entry into more sophisticated mathematical reasoning.

SERIAL MEMORY PROBLEMS IN MATHEMATICS BY CHILDREN WITH SLI

Problems with serial memory in children with SLI can be seen in their impaired performance on mathematical tasks that require fast retrieval of numbers in a specific order (Fazio, 1994b, 1996). Fazio (1994b) examined the counting abilities of 20 preschool children with SLI compared with 20 language-matched and 20 mental age–matched peers without SLI. To detect the nature of the difficulties that children with SLI exhibited in counting, the investigators had the subjects participate in a series of counting tasks. Despite displaying knowledge of many rules associated with counting, preschool children with SLI displayed marked difficulty in rote counting, displayed a limited repertoire of number terms and therefore miscounted sets of objects. It appeared that a lack of the correct sequence of counting words prevented them from correctly counting the sets of objects. For example, if the set size was not larger than the set of correctly ordered number words that they could recite, they often gave the correct response. In other words, the primary difference between the counting abilities of children with SLI and their cognitively matched peers was knowledge of the correct sequence of number words. These findings suggest that such children have a specific difficulty with the rote serial aspect of learning number words. Rote sequence problems of a similar nature were found in many children at risk for SLI (Fazio, Naremore, & Connell, 1996).

The children with SLI that participated in the above counting study also were seen in a two-year follow-up study (Fazio, 1996). Fourteen first- and second-grade children with SLI were compared with two comparison groups of children without SLI. There were 15 children in the typically developing mental age–matched group and 16 children in the language-matched group. The children participated in a series of tasks that examined rule knowledge of numbers with actual mathematical performance. Despite displaying knowledge of many conceptual aspects of numbers such as counting plates of cookies to decide which plate has "more," children with SLI displayed marked difficulty performing tasks that required an immediate response such as rote counting to 50, counting by 10s, or reciting numerals backward from 20. Moreover, these children did much better on numerical tasks that allowed them to use actual objects to count and on math problems that did not require them to exceed the sequence of numbers that they knew well. These findings offer further evidence that automatic retrieval of rote serial material is particularly cumbersome for children with SLI.

It is important to note that children with SLI did make steady progress in their mathematical abilities over the two-year period. Despite delays they exhibited with respect to number sequences, they had learned a great deal about numbers. Their knowledge about the rules of counting and their understanding of the usefulness of counting for solving addition problems were strengths for them. When children with SLI were given sufficient time to count aloud or to use their fingers, their performance on addition and subtraction problems surpassed that of their language-matched peers. Furthermore, they were good at counting actual objects to add sets and using their fingers to solve addition problems. In other words, in contrast to their rote memory for numerical material, SLI children's general knowledge of many of the rules related to numbers was not delayed.

The pattern of results from the follow-up study and the original counting investigation suggests that two types of knowledge of mathematics are slow to develop in children with SLI. They fail to produce number words in the proper sequence and they have difficulty recalling certain memorized material such as math facts. Both problems suggest that children with SLI may be particularly vulnerable to failure when storing or retrieving phonological forms. Recall that at first children learn to count as a chant—"one, two, three." The number words are not linked semantically with a referent. Therefore, its primary feature is the phonological form of the words. If children with SLI do not have adequate temporary storage, the process of constructing stable long-term memory is hindered. In a similar vein, successful retrieval of words requires an accurate initial phonetic representation and an efficient short-term storage of this presentation (Liberman, 1982).

Difficulty with rapid solutions for simple addition and subtraction problems was characteristic of children with SLI in the Fazio (1996) follow-up study. Rather than retrieving facts, these children appeared to use counting procedures to calculate answers. If they did not exhaust their knowledge of counting words, they were successful with this technique. In fact, many of their classmates were using the same simple counting strategies to solve problems. However, the literature on mathematical abilities suggests that by third or fourth grade increased efficiency (i.e., speed) and automaticity are required. For example, the time needed to do addition problems is closely related to counting rates for younger children but not for older children (Ashcraft, 1985). An inability to solve simple math problems rapidly and accurately is cited as a frequent problem for fourth- to sixth-grade children with learning disabilities (e.g., Cawley, Miller, & School, 1987). This follow-up study suggests that the antecedents of this problem in children also are seen for those just starting elementary school.

SERIAL MEMORY AND PRESCHOOLERS' KNOWLEDGE OF NURSERY RHYMES

There is now a substantial body of evidence suggesting that phonological awareness skills are related to reading ability (see Blachman, 1994; Catts, 1989; Goswami & Bryant, 1990, for reviews). However, there has been considerable debate concerning the role of phonological awareness as a precursor to reading. Some evidence suggests that attention to the sound structure such as rhyme before formal reading instruction is an important precursor to reading (e.g., Bryant, Bradley, Maclean, & Crossland, 1989; Maclean et al., 1987). For example, a relationship has been observed between children's early knowledge of nursery rhymes such as Baa, Baa, Black Sheep and first- and second-grade reading performance (Bryant et al., 1989; Maclean et al., 1987). These studies suggest that knowledge of rhyme and alliteration help children understand that reading is based—in part—on the alphabetic principle that letters represent spoken language at the phonemic level. Children with this type of phonological awareness also are more likely to understand that alphabetic writing represents the sounds of spoken language as well as the meaning (e.g., Adams, 1990). However, other evidence suggests that experience in reading leads to phonological awareness (e.g., Morais, Cluyens, Alegria, & Content, 1986). Bryant, Maclean, Bradley, and Crossland (1990) help clarify this discussion by distinguishing between simpler phonological skills (e.g., rhyme and alliteration tasks) that precede reading and more difficult phonological tasks (e.g., phoneme manipulation tasks) that develop with reading.

Studies showing a relationship between general sound sensitivity and later reading performance suggest that valuable information for the beginner reader is contained in informal linguistic routines such as nursery rhymes, finger plays, and songs. These rote sequences are often learned as part of the child's home or preschool classroom experiences (Maclean et al., 1987). This research suggests that children gain important information about rhyme and alliteration from memorizing such poems in which the prosodic features of the poem stress the shared sounds in words. Nursery rhymes and poetry naturally emphasize phonological structures without explicitly requiring the child to understand metalinguistic concepts related to the organization of language (Gathercole & Baddeley, 1993). Apparently, this early information is then used as evidence when children begin to use developing metalinguistic (conscious) awareness of initial and final sounds in words and syllable and word segmentation (van Kleeck, 1995). Findings of this nature are exciting because they suggest that preschool children with language learning difficulties could be exposed to nursery rhymes as preschoolers and reap the benefits of such learning when they start an organized reading instruction program.

KNOWLEDGE OF NURSERY RHYMES IN PRESCHOOLERS WITH SLI

Given the strong relationship between early rhyming and phonological awareness abilities and later reading abilities (e.g., Bryant et al., 1989; Maclean et al., 1987), it is important to understand the nature of the difficulty children with SLI face with rhymes and to develop techniques to help their learning and recall of poems. Research by Fazio (in press) provides evidence that preschool children with SLI have difficulty memorizing Mother Goose rhymes and songs. In the first study in this series, 10 low-income kindergarten children with SLI were compared with 10 low-income peers on three rote linguistic sequence tasks: reciting common nursery rhymes, reciting the alphabet, and rote counting. Compared with their low-income, age-matched classmates without SLI, children with SLI displayed poorer performance on rote counting. Their performance also was severely delayed when asked to recite Mother Goose nursery rhymes.

The second study, Fazio (in press), examined the learning and retention of nursery rhymes in young low-income children with and without SLI during six weeks of classroom instruction. Eight 4- and 5-year-old low-income children with SLI and eight of their low-income age-matched classmates were taught five novel Mother Goose rhymes during a large group classroom activity. The teacher held up a large picture depicting the events of the rhyme. The teacher recited the rhyme once and asked the children to recite the rhyme with her. Children were tested before and after the intervention on their ability to recite nursery rhymes and on their ability to detect rhyme. Compared with their peers, children with SLI had difficulty repeating the nursery rhymes even after daily classroom exposure for the six-week period. There is some evidence that increased practice would help performance in children with SLI. For example, in study one of the Fazio (in press) research described earlier, 7 of 10 low-income kindergarten children with SLI and 10 of 10 children without a language impairment could sing the alphabet song. (The children's best performance of two trials was used in this measure.) The kindergarten children had been enrolled in public school for one semester, and their classroom teachers reported that singing or reciting the alphabet was a daily classroom activity.

In the final study in this series, Fazio (1994a) taught 48 preschool children with and without SLI a new poem under four conditions: with or without hand motions that accompanied the rhyme and with or without an accompanying melody. The 32 children without SLI in the study showed no learning style preferences; they learned the rhyme in all conditions and could recite most of the poem two days later. As expected, the 16 preschool children with SLI had difficulty learning the poem in all conditions. However, their recall of the poem was much better in the condition that had accompanying hand motions. It appears that the hand motions were used as cues for each section of the poem. Although the use of a melody did not appear to facilitate learning or retrieval of the poem, the children learned a new melody (to control for prior knowledge). Therefore, it is not known if using a familiar melody such as the tune to "Happy Birthday" also would help retrieval. Some evidence that familiar songs facilitate rote memory was gained from the kindergarten nursery rhyme knowledge study (Fazio, 1994a). In that study, all but three children in the SLI group correctly sang the alphabet song. It appears that at least one song was well learned by kindergarten children with SLI in that study.

ASSESSMENT ISSUES

Knowledge of rote linguistic sequences such as counting may be an effective screening tool for identifying children at risk for language-related academic problems in school. For children with SLI, timed performance on tasks requiring rote linguistic memory has been poor. Several studies have shown similar problems with rapid automatized naming (e.g., Denckla & Rudel, 1976) and confrontational naming (e.g., Wolf & Goodglass, 1986). It may be that reaction time and timed performances of counting to 100, counting by 10s, counting backward from 20, and number facts (and tasks of a similar nature) reveal problems that are not seen when time is not an issue. For example, in the Fazio study (1996) response times of greater than three seconds were common for first- and second-grade children with SLI. However, their cognitively matched peers often answered with no noticeable delay. A standardized test that uses timed tests of word finding can be found in the Test of Word Finding (German, 1986).

Timed tasks of this nature might play an important role in an assessment battery designed to identify children who have or who are at risk for having language learning problems in elementary school.

A clue to whether preschoolers will have one avenue of access to sound similarity (both initial and final sounds) is their ability to recite (knowledge of) nursery rhymes and poems. This is a simple task to assess. In the studies described earlier, children viewed a page from a Mother Goose book (with the text removed) and were asked to say the rhyme. One measure of rhyme knowledge, therefore, is the percentage of the rhyme recited correctly. However, looking at the general pattern seen in the literature on rhyme knowledge, children generally fell into three categories: (1) those who knew the rhyme well, (2) those who knew parts of the rhyme, or (3) those who showed no knowledge of the rhyme. Researchers such as Bryant et al. (1989) have used these three categories rather than percentage of the rhyme recited correctly as a grading scale to judge rhyme knowledge.

A third assessment item of interest would be a child's ability to learn a new rhyme. One measure of such knowledge would be the number of words correctly recited. This also could be represented as a percentage correctly recited. An additional measure could be the number of trials needed to learn each line of the poem. For example, Fazio et al. (1996) used the following procedure to compute knowledge of a new rhyme. The second-grade children were taught an eight-line novel poem. First, the children individually repeated each line of the poem after the adult said the line in order for a minimum of four times for each line. Then each child was asked to recite the poem. If the child could repeat the poem with three or fewer prompts from the adult, the poem was considered learned. A prompt consisted of the next word in the poem. Then the child performed an intervening task such as drawing with markers and chatting with the adult for 10 minutes. The child was asked to recite the poem again. The 11 children without SLI in this study took, on average, 40 repetitions to recite the entire poem without help, whereas the 12 children in the SLI group took, on average, 54 repetitions to recite the poem. Another measure of rhyme knowledge was the percentage correctly recited after a 10-minute delay. This percentage was calculated by counting the number of words correctly recited divided by the total number of words in the poem. Children without SLI could recite, on average, 77% of the poem with three or fewer adult prompts. Children with SLI could recite, on average, 54% of the poem with three or fewer adult prompts.

MATHEMATICS INTERVENTION ISSUES

How can young children's performance on rote serial tasks be improved? Research suggests that the key to automaticity is practice (Logan, 1988). In children without SLI, practice routinely serves to strengthen rote knowledge, and it is the basic mechanism used to explain expertise in addition and subtraction (Ashcraft, 1985). Therefore, one way to help young children with SLI would be to provide more opportunities to count—counting chants, games, and songs, and counting actual objects.

However, given that counting strategies alone are not sufficient for later mathematical problem solving and given that counting may not be a strength for children with SLI, some systematic approach to help children with SLI is needed to produce rapid number sequences and number fact retrieval. Several intervention programs have been proposed to increase automaticity of math facts in children with learning disabilities (LDs). One technique that Hasselbring, Gain, and Bransford (1987) suggest is the use of computer games to drill math facts. They report success with this method for providing the practice needed to achieve automaticity. It may be the case that classic rote drill of math facts will be an effective way of promoting automaticity of math facts for children with SLI.

The current literature on mathematics instruction also stresses the pitfalls of using only drill and practice activities to strengthen mathematical performance. For example, the National Council of Teachers of Mathematics (1989) has condemned the current practice of teaching mathematics with a focus on calculation. Instead, they suggest that math be embedded in a real-world context, and calculation should be used as a tool for solving real-world problems. Therefore, they advocate repetitive meaning-based instruction in mathematics. This intervention strategy fits quite nicely with many models of early language intervention. In such models, everyday activities between parents and children (or teachers and children) are used as natural informal teaching situations. Incorporating more opportunities to count for a specific purpose such as counting out the number of forks needed for the table could easily be adapted into everyday home and classroom routines.

Several researchers including Baroody and Ginsburg (1986), Parmar and Cawley (1991), and Scheid (1990) suggest that metacognitive strategies may enhance basic number fact knowledge. Metacognitive strategies refer to techniques that assist in "thinking through" problems. Research on children without SLI has shown that children who are successful with math facts use "thinking strategies" as a memory aid (Goldman, 1989). It may be that techniques suggested by German (1992) such as self-cuing to retrieve a missing word also may be effective intervention strategies. Such techniques are described in more detail in the next section.

It remains an empirical question as to which combination of intervention strategies such as drill in counting and math facts, word-retrieval strategies, repetitive meaning-based instruction, or metacognitive strategies to aid recall will be the most effective combination for children with SLI.

RHYME INTERVENTION STRATEGIES

It may be the case that children with SLI need a more direct teaching strategy than the informal routines used with preschoolers without SLI. What is not clear, however, is how to offer children with SLI more practice in reciting rhymes. Do children need to engage in reciting the rhymes aloud, or is listening to the rhymes for an extended period sufficient input? At the least, work by Fazio (1994a, in press) suggests that children with SLI need significantly more practice time to learn nursery rhymes.

The literature on word-finding intervention provides strategies that may facilitate storage and recall of rote linguistic sequences. However, it is unclear whether techniques designed to help storage of individual words also are effective in storing and retrieving rote sequences. Unlike storing labels for objects and actions, in which a richer knowledge base of the target word's semantic meaning can serve as an aid to recall, memorized lines of text are most likely learned as partially or completely unanalyzed phrases. However, breaking the nursery rhymes into smaller segments (e.g., one line at a time) such as saying one line then repeating the line with the child may enhance memorization. Practice combined with visual imagery may be another effective way to memorize such material. For example, visual imagery helped word retrieval in children with word-finding problems (e.g., McGregor & Leonard, 1989; Wing, 1990). Acting out the activities in the rhyme or viewing pictures of the rhyme as a series of action sequences may help store the rhyme as smaller elements that have a visual component (German, 1992). Fazio (1994a) found that including hand motions that match the actions of the rhyme helped storage and retrieval of a novel nursery rhyme. Adding a melody such as the alphabet song appeared to help children with SLI remember the rote sequence (Fazio, in press).

Both these techniques introduce an additional modality on which to store such sequences.

There is convincing evidence that the metalinguistic abilities of children with SLI are delayed (e.g., Kamhi, 1987; van Kleeck, 1994). Given this information, practice with nursery rhymes alone is not likely to be sufficient intervention. Therefore, games and activities specifically designed to stimulate phonological awareness need to be incorporated into the preschool classroom experiences of children with SLI (e.g., Fey, Catts, & Larrivee, 1995; Gillam & van Kleeck, Chapter 5). There are now several studies in the literature that document success in stimulating typically developing preschool children to attend to the phonological patterns of language (e.g., Bradley & Bryant, 1983; Lundberg, Frost, & Petersen, 1988). In addition, two recent studies by Warrick, Rubin, and Rowe-Walsh (1993) and O'Connor, Jenkins, Leicester, and Slocum (1993) have focused on phonological awareness intervention in children with language learning difficulties. This type of intervention has ranged in length from six weeks to nine months. In such studies, the route to phonological sensitivity is not through children's knowledge of rote linguistic sequences such as nursery rhymes, but through a series of activities designed to increase the awareness of the sound patterns found in the language.

•   •   •

Given the clear relationship between rote counting and success in arithmetic, such sequences need to be overlearned and highly accessible for the arithmetic skills in children with SLI to advance. Given the apparent relationship among early nursery rhyme knowledge, phonological awareness abilities, and later reading performance, it is equally important to understand the nature of the difficulty children with SLI face with reciting rhymes and to develop techniques to facilitate their learning and recall of poems (along with other techniques that foster phonological awareness). Therefore, assessing young children's rote linguistic knowledge is an important component of language assessment. These rote sequences lend themselves to everyday parent and classroom teacher activities. As interventionists, clinicians and teachers have the opportunity to teach these rote sequences in meaningful contexts such as having a child count the number of cookies needed for snack or sending home a tape of the class singing finger plays and nursery rhymes. Parents and teachers need to be informed about the important role that counting and nursery rhymes can play in young children's experiences and the need to incorporate counting and reciting rhymes throughout young children's everyday experiences.

REFERENCES

Adams, M. (1990). *Beginning to read: Thinking and learning about print*. Cambridge, MA: MIT Press.

Ashcraft, M.H. (1985). The development of mental arithmetic: A chronometric approach. *Developmental Review, 2*, 213–236.

Baddeley, A.D. (1986). *Working memory*. Oxford, England: Clarendon Press.

Baroody, A.J., & Ginsburg, H.P. (1986). The relationship between initial meaningful and mechanical knowledge of arithmetic. In J. Hiebert (Ed.), *Conceptual and procedural knowledge: The case of mathematics* (pp. 75–112). Hillsdale, NJ: Lawrence Erlbaum.

Bates, E., Bretherton, I., & Snyder, L. (1988). From first words to grammar: Individual differences and dissociable mechanisms. Cambridge, England: Cambridge University Press.

Blachman, B.A. (1994). Early literacy acquisition: The role of phonological awareness. In G. Wallach & K. Butler (Eds.), *Language learning disabilities in school-age children and adolescents: Some principles and applications* (pp. 271–287). New York: Macmillan.

Bradley, L., & Bryant, P. (1983). Categorizing sounds and learning to read: A usual connection. *Nature, 30*, 419–421.

Bryant, P.E., Bradley, L., Maclean, M., & Crossland, J. (1989). Nursery rhymes, phonological skills and reading. *Journal of Child Language, 16*, 407–428.

Bryant, P.E., Maclean, M., Bradley, L., & Crossland, J. (1990). Rhyme and alliteration, phoneme detection, and learning to read. *Developmental Psychology, 26*, 429–438.

Carpenter, T.P., & Moser, J.M. (1984). The acquisition of addition and subtraction: Concepts in grades one through three. *Journal of Research in Mathematics Education, 15*, 179–202.

Catts, H. (1989). Phonological processing deficits and reading disabilities. In A. Kamhi & H. Catts (Eds.), *Reading disabilities: A developmental language perspective* (pp. 101–132). Austin, TX: PRO-ED.

Cawley, J.F., Miller, J.H., & School, B.A. (1987). A brief inquiry of arithmetic word problem solving among learning disabled secondary students. *Learning Disabilities Focus, 2*, 87–93.

Denckla, M., & Rudel, R. (1976). "Rapid automatized naming": Dyslexia differentiated from other learning disabilities. *Neuropsychologia, 14*, 471–479.

Fazio, B.B. (1994a). *The impact of multimodal learning on SLI children's phonological memory*. Paper presented at the annual meeting of American Speech-Language-Hearing Association, New Orleans, LA.

Fazio, B.B. (1994b). Counting abilities of children with specific language impairment: A comparison of oral and gestural tasks. *Journal of Speech and Hearing Research, 37*, 358–368.

Fazio, B.B. (1996). Mathematical abilities of children with specific language impairment. *Journal of Speech and Hearing Research, 39*, 1–11.

Fazio, B.B. (in press). Memory for rote linguistic routines and sensitivity to rhyme: A comparison of low income children with and without specific language impairment. *Applied Psycholinguistics.*

Fazio, B.B., Naremore, R.C., & Connell, P.C. (1996). Tracking children at risk for specific language impairment: A three year longitudinal study. *Journal of Speech and Hearing Research, 39*, 52–63.

Fey, M.E., Catts, H.W., & Larrivee, L.S. (1995). Preparing preschoolers for the academic and social challenges of school. In M.E. Fey, J. Windsor, & S.F. Warren (Eds.), *Language intervention: Preschool through the elementary years* (pp. 3–38). Baltimore: Brookes.

Fuson, K.C. (1988). *Children's counting and concepts of number.* New York: Springer-Verlag.

Fuson, K.C., Pergament, G.G., & Lyons, B.C. (1985). Children's conformity to the cardinality rule as a function of set size and counting accuracy. *Child Development, 56*, 1429–1439.

Gathercole, S.F., & Baddeley, A.D. (1990). Phonological memory deficits in language disordered children: Is there a causal connection? *Journal of Memory and Language, 29*, 336–360.

Gathercole, S.F., & Baddeley, A.D. (1993). *Working memory and language.* Hove, East Sussex, England: Lawrence Erlbaum.

German, D.J. (1986). *National College of Education Test of Word Finding (TWF).* Chicago: Riverside.

German, D.J. (1992). Word-finding intervention for children and adolescents. *Topics in Language Disorders, 13*, 33–50.

Gillam, R.B., Cowan, N., & Day, L.S. (1995). Sequential memory in children with and without language impairment. *Journal of Speech and Hearing Research, 38*, 393–402.

Goldman, S.R. (1989). Strategy instruction in mathematics. *Learning Disability Quarterly, 89*, 43–53.

Goswami, C., & Bryant, P.E. (1990). *Phonological skill and learning to read.* London: Lawrence Erlbaum.

Hasselbring, T.S., Gain, L.I., & Bransford, J.D. (1987). Effective mathematics instruction: Developing automaticity. *Teaching Exceptional Children, 19*, 30–33.

Just, M.A., & Carpenter, P.A. (1992). A capacity theory of comprehension: Individual differences in working memory. *Psychological Review, 99*, 122–149.

Kail, R. (1990). *The development of memory in children* (3rd ed.). New York: W.H. Freeman.

Kail, R., & Leonard, L.B. (1986). Word-finding abilities in language-impaired children. *ASHA Monographs, 25*, 1–85.

Kamhi, A. (1987). Metalinguistic abilities in language-impaired children. *Topics in Language Disorders, 7*, 1–12.

Kirchner, D., & Klatzky, R. (1985). Verbal rehearsal and memory in language-disordered children. *Journal of Speech and Hearing Research, 28*, 556–565.

Lahey, M. (1988). *Language disorders and language development.* New York: Macmillan.

Liberman, I.Y. (1982). A language-oriented view of reading and its disabilities. In H. Mykelbust (Ed.), *Progress in learning disabilities* (Vol. 5, pp. 81–101). New York: Grune & Stratton.

Logan, G.D. (1988). Toward an instance theory of automatization. *Psychological Review, 95*, 492–502.

Lundberg, I., Frost, J., & Petersen, O. (1988). Effects of an extensive program for stimulating phonological awareness in preschool children. *Reading Research Quarterly, 23*, 263–284.

Maclean, M., Bryant, P.E., & Bradley, L. (1987). Rhymes, nursery rhymes, and reading in early childhood. *Merrill-Palmer Quarterly, 33*, 255–282.

McGregor, K.K., & Leonard, L.B. (1989). Facilitating word-finding skills of language-impaired children. *Journal of Speech and Hearing Disorders, 54*, 141–147.

Morais, J., Cluyens, M., Alegria, J., & Content, A. (1986). Speech mediated retention in dyslexia. *Perceptual and Motor Skills, 62*, 119–126.

National Council of Teachers of Mathematics. (1989). *Curriculum and evaluation standards for school mathematics.* Reston, VA: Author.

O'Connor, R.E., Jenkins, J.R., Leicester, N., & Slocum, T.A. (1993). Teaching phonological awareness to young children with learning disabilities. *Exceptional Children, 59*, 532–546.

Parmar, R.S., & Cawley, J.F. (1991). Challenging the routine and passivity that characterize arithmetic instruction for children with mild handicaps. *Research and Special Education, 12*, 23–32, 43.

Peters, A. (1983). *The units of language acquisition.* Cambridge, England: Cambridge University Press.

Resnick, L.B. (1983). A developmental theory of number understanding. In H. Ginsburg (Ed.), *The development of children's mathematical thinking* (pp. 210–224). New York: Academic Press.

Scheid, K. (1990). *Cognitive-based methods for teaching mathematics to students with learning problems.* Columbus, OH: LINC Resources.

Sininger, Y.S., Klatzky, R.L., & Kirchner, D.M. (1989). Memory scanning speed in language-disordered children. *Journal of Speech and Hearing Research, 32*, 289–297.

van Kleeck, A. (1994). Metalinguistic development. In G.P. Wallach & K. Butler (Eds.), *Language learning disabilities in school-age children and adolescents.* New York: Macmillan.

van Kleeck, A. (1995). Emphasizing form and meaning separately in prereading and early reading instruction. *Topics in Language Disorders, 16,* 27–49.

Warrick, N., Rubin, H., & Rowe-Walsh, S. (1993). Phoneme awareness in language-delayed children: Comparative studies and intervention. *Annals of Dyslexia, 43,* 153–173.

Wing, C.S. (1990). A preliminary investigation of generalization to untrained words following two treatments of children's word-finding problems. *Language, Speech and Hearing Services in Schools, 21,* 151–156.

Wolf, M., & Goodglass, A. (1986). Dyslexia, dysnomia and lexical retrieval: A longitudinal investigation. *Brain and Language, 28,* 154–168.

5

Phonological Awareness Training and Short-Term Working Memory: Clinical Implications

Ronald B. Gillam and Anne van Kleeck

Children with language impairment and learning disabilities have difficulty with a wide range of working memory and phonological awareness tasks. Phonological working memory—the ability to process and hold verbal information in immediate attention—has been shown to be related to spoken language development and reading. Similarly, numerous studies have demonstrated that phonological awareness—the ability to consciously reflect on and manipulate the sound component of language—is related to early reading and spelling achievement (e.g., Lundberg, Frost, & Petersen, 1988; Torgesen, Morgan, & Davis, 1992). Some investigators have advised clinicians to target phonological working memory in therapy (Gathercole & Baddeley, 1993; Montgomery, Chapter 2). Likewise, many ideas for applications of phonological awareness research for working with young children who have language delays have been published in issues of *Topics in Language Disorders* (e.g., Blachman, 1991; Jenkins & Bowen, 1994; van Kleeck, 1990, 1995).

Clinicians may wonder whether they should focus on phonological working memory, phonological awareness, neither, or both in their intervention. It could easily be argued that there are not enough data to answer

This work was supported by research grant number 5 K08 DC 00086-03 from the National Institute on Deafness and Other Communication Disorders, National Institutes of Health.

Top Lang Disord 1996;17(1):72–81

this question. However, unlike researchers, clinicians do not have the luxury of waiting until data are in before generating answers to difficult questions. The best approach to making clinical decisions may be to combine theoretical and empirical information to arrive at a course of action that makes sense given the available knowledge. That is precisely what the authors attempt to do in this chapter. Based on theories of the relationship between phonological awareness and phonological working memory, a theory of intervention, and data from a recent efficacy study, the authors suggest that phonological awareness constitutes a valid focus for intervention. Furthermore, the authors believe targeting phonological awareness will affect early literacy development as well as certain aspects of phonological working memory.

This chapter reviews current thinking about phonological working memory, phonological awareness, and the relationship between these processes. There are two aspects of phonological working memory—phonological coding and phonological recoding—that appear to be key elements in this relationship and in the relationship of both skills to early reading development. The authors' approach to language intervention will be discussed, and a rationale will be offered for focusing on phonological awareness rather than phonological working memory. Finally, the results of an efficacy study in which preschoolers with language impairments were trained in phonological awareness skills are summarized.

PHONOLOGICAL WORKING MEMORY

As in Cowan's work (1995, Chapter 1), the term *phonological working memory* here refers to an aspect of memory that functions as more than just a memory store. Phonological working memory is a process in which verbal information is coded and kept immediately accessible through activation and reactivation operations. Research suggests that there are several aspects within phonological working memory. Initially, acoustic, temporal, and sequential aspects of sounds are represented in a sensory trace that lasts for a short amount of time before fading (Cowan, 1995). This sensory trace is translated into a stable phonological representation through a process called *phonological coding*. When working memory processes translate visual information such as printed or pictured words into phonological representations, the process is referred to as *phonological recoding*

(Gathercole & Baddeley, 1990, 1993). Finally, phonological representations—or phonological codes—are stored together with meaning representations in long-term memory (e.g., Dollaghan, 1987). These representations can be kept immediately accessible in attention through rehearsal.

Phonological working memory is often measured by word and nonword span tasks. Memory span is considered to be the longest list of words (or nonwords) that can be repeated without error. In word span tasks (including digit span), learners repeat lists of words spoken by an examiner. Nonword span tasks work the same way, except the stimulus lists are composed of phonologically viable nonwords rather than real words. Nonword recall tasks are thought to be sensitive measures of phonological coding abilities because the nature of the stimuli minimizes potential top-down influences of lexical knowledge, whereas word span task performance is more confounded by such top-down influences (Gathercole & Baddeley, 1993).

Phonological awareness

Phonological awareness is a general term used to refer to the conscious knowledge that words in language are composed of various units of sound. The synonymous term *metaphonology* reminds one that awareness of the sound component of language is but one manifestation of a more general language awareness or metalinguistic skill.

Phonological awareness can occur on syllabic, subsyllabic, and phonemic levels. Awareness of syllabic sound units is generally assessed by having children segment words into component syllables. The subsyllabic units intermediate between syllables and phonemes are called *onsets* and *rimes* (see Treiman, 1992, for example). "The onset is the initial consonant or consonant cluster of a syllable, and the rime is the remainder of the syllable. It always contains a vowel, and optionally contains a final consonant or consonant cluster" (van Kleeck, 1995, p. 35). Children demonstrate awareness of onset and rime sound units in language when they recognize or generate rhymes, because words that rhyme generally have different onsets while sharing a rime (as in *fox* and *box*). Awareness of individual phonemes and their sequence is typically assessed by having children identify sounds within words (e.g., "What is the first sound in *ball*?" "What word starts with the sound /d/?").

Developmental changes in phonological representation and phonological awareness

It is often assumed that phonemes are the phonological units that are represented and stored in memory, but there is some indication that the unit of representation changes during development. For example, Fowler (1991) suggests that the first 50 words are stored as holistic patterns or whole word shapes. As the child's lexicon expands, the scope of representation may narrow, giving salience to syllabic units first and then to subsyllabic and phonemic units later. The implication is that phoneme-level representations of speech gradually emerge during the preschool years. This developmental sequence appears to parallel the development of phonological awareness. Children are first able to isolate entire words within sentences, then syllables within words, and finally phonemes within words (e.g., Fox & Routh, 1975). Recent work by Treiman (1992) indicates that awareness of the subsyllabic units of onset and rime also emerges before phonemic awareness. Indeed, young preschoolers will spontaneously produce rhymes (Dowker, 1989) and three-year-olds can detect rhymes in experimental tasks (Maclean, Bryant, & Bradley, 1987). Because rhyming is a spontaneously occurring phonological awareness skill, and because it is present in many preschool games and books, it may be an important training target in intervention designed to foster phonological awareness. This is the approach taken in an intervention study with preschoolers with language impairments that will be discussed later.

The relationship between phonological awareness and phonological working memory

Phonological working memory is necessary for performing phonological awareness tasks. This is because the phonological coding and recoding processes that are inherent in phonological working memory play an important role in phonological awareness. When children are asked to identify the first sound in the word *ball*, for example, they translate the acoustic trace of /bal/ into a stable phonological representation. At some point in development, this representation probably contains information about specific phonemes and their sequences. For children to correctly respond to the request, they must keep the representation active in working memory long enough to analyze the phonemes in order and to determine that the first phoneme is /b/.

The development of word recognition in early reading involves a combination of phonological working memory and phonological analysis skills. There appear to be two primary forms of word recognition. In an indirect route, sometimes referred to as *sounding out,* readers use their knowledge of grapheme–phoneme correspondences to recode visual letters or multiletter patterns into sequences of sounds. The ability to recode print requires insight into what is called the *alphabetic principle*—knowing that letters stand for individual sounds in spoken words. This insight involves the integration of both alphabetic knowledge (knowing letter names, letter shapes, and corresponding sounds) and phoneme awareness (knowing how to analyze or synthesize the sounds). When sequences of sounds are coded, children search their mental lexicon for words that match the phonological sequences (Adams, 1990). In a direct route, sometimes referred to as *sight reading,* readers automatically access pronunciation and meaning when they see words that they have read many times before. Experienced readers tend to read directly (by sight), except when they encounter conceptually difficult material or words that are unknown (Samuels, 1994).

In the indirect route, phonological coding and recoding processes enable readers to bond sequences of orthographic representations with sequences of phonemic representations in memory (Perfetti, 1992). Later, these bonds serve as access routes for direct connections between letter sequences and their corresponding phonological, semantic, syntactic, and spelling representations (Ehri, 1992, 1994). It is in indirect reading that the phonological coding and recoding processes in working memory and phonological awareness most obviously interact to support word recognition.

LANGUAGE INTERVENTION

Clinicians who do not believe in teaching aspects of language form separate from language content and use would be unlikely to focus on either phonological working memory or phonological awareness targets in language intervention. The authors believe early language intervention should foster social–interactive uses of language in pragmatically relevant contexts. However, the authors also believe that preschool-age and school-age children can benefit from a temporary focus on particular aspects of language form separate from language content and/or use (Gillam, McFadden, & van Kleeck, 1995; van Kleeck, 1995). Phonological working memory and phonological awareness are two examples of just such form-oriented intervention targets. Intervention in these areas seems warranted because they are important precursors to decoding print and because children with language impairments frequently present difficulties in both areas. Clinicians who share the authors' general philosophical orientation to language intervention could reasonably wonder whether to target working memory skills, phonological awareness skills, or both in conjunction with therapy that focuses on interactions among language form, content, and use.

It could be argued that phonological working memory is the more powerful intervention target because working memory relates to a wide variety of language skills, including language comprehension, vocabulary development, metalinguistics, and decoding print. Targeting memory skills in intervention was popular in the 1960s and 1970s as one aspect of a broader approach to language intervention that Bloom and Lahey (1978) and Lahey (1988) have referred to as the *specific-abilities model*. Studies of children with learning disabilities have consistently shown that—with training—performance on memory tasks can be improved. However, the authors have yet to find a study demonstrating that memory training results in improved language or literacy.

Phonological awareness is related to only one skill—decoding print— and for this reason might seem to be a less powerful target. However, unlike working memory training, training in phonological awareness has a direct impact on prereading, early reading, or spelling ability in nearly all the studies to date (e.g., Ball & Blachman, 1991; Bradley & Bryant, 1985; Byrne & Fielding-Barnsley, 1991; Fox & Routh, 1984; Lundberg et al., 1988; Williams, 1980).

Given the consistently positive outcomes of phonological awareness training and the critical importance of early reading for academic, social, and vocational success, the authors decided to investigate the impact of training phonological awareness in preschool children with language impairment. Because the authors suspected that phonological awareness depends on phonological working memory skills, as discussed earlier, they included pre- and postintervention measures of working memory in the design. This allowed the authors to test the hypothesis that phonological working memory underlies phonological awareness skills, following Brady's (1991) suggestion that "the consequences of a limited working capacity . . . may make it more difficult to discover and master meta-phonological skills" (pp. 130–131). As such, children with better working memories at the outset (and hence a better phonological coding and recoding) should benefit most from phonological awareness training. However, it may be that training in phonological awareness could enhance phonological working memory because it would give the child practice in phonological coding. The data allowed the authors to explore both of these possibilities.

The phonological awareness training that the authors developed consisted of two stages. During the first stage, preschool-age children with language impairment were taught rhyming tasks twice weekly for one semester and phoneme awareness tasks twice weekly for the second semester. The authors started with rhyming, rather than word and syllable segmentation, for the following reasons. Word segmentation can be accomplished semantically rather than phonologically because words are meaningful units. Thus, word segmentation did not seem a viable starting point for phonological awareness training. Children develop the ability to deal with the subsyllabic units of rime at about the same time that they segment words into syllables. The authors thought it would be most efficient to begin phonological awareness training with the smallest phonological unit that children could handle successfully (i.e., the onset and rime units used in rhyming).

Other studies of phonological awareness have included a rhyme (or "rime") level of training. Lundberg and colleagues (1988) started with rhyming, but then moved to word segmentation and then syllables. Because rhymes already focus the child's attention at the subsyllabic level of onset and rime, the additional steps of words and syllables used in Lundberg and colleagues' study seemed unnecessary to the authors. Fox and Routh (1984) trained onset and rime segmentation and blending, but did not move on to the phoneme level. Bradley and Bryant's (1985) study began with rhyming and then included phoneme awareness in a second step that focused on sound/letter correspondences. However, phoneme awareness was not trained independently before it was incorporated with letters and letter sounds. In the authors' study, they began with rhyming tasks and then moved on to the phoneme level, following Adams' (1990) conclusion that "exploitation of onsets and rimes could well provide the key to unlocking phonemic awareness" (p. 318).

The intervention study

Gillam and van Kleeck (in press) trained 16 preschool-age children with developmental speech and language disorders on phonological awareness tasks for a period of nine months. The children attended a private school for children with communication disorders. Eight of the children (mean age = 4;1) had been placed in a preschool I classroom. The other eight children (mean age = 5;0) had been placed in a preschool II classroom. Both classes met for three hours each day. A group of older children with speech and language impairments from the same school (mean age = 6;0) were tested at the beginning of the year, but did not receive phonological awareness training. Including this control group enabled the researchers to compare the performance of younger children with language impairments who had received phonological awareness training with older children with language impairments who had not.

Rhyme intervention

During the fall semester, two graduate student clinicians in speech-language pathology conducted rhyming activities with small groups of children who rotated through a classroom rhyming center. Children attended a rhyming center for 15 minutes twice each week. Rhyming center activities focused on five rhyme pairs each week. Children were led through a series of increasingly difficult rhyming activities with each set of rhyme pairs, progressing from recognition, to imitation, to identification, to judgment, and finally to rhyme creation. In addition, classroom teachers (who also were speech-language pathologists) read aloud every day from a rhyming book (e.g., *Itchy, Itchy Chicken Pox*, Maccarone & Lewin, 1992) that contained the target rhyming word pairs. Picture cards and a "game board" also were created for the rhyme pairs.

In the first rhyming center each week, graduate student clinicians read a book aloud that contained at least five target rhyme pairs. For *Itchy, Itchy Chicken Pox*, these rhyme pairs were *pox/socks, toes/nose, now/ow, four/more*, and *spots/lots*. Clinicians told the children that the book would be read aloud in class daily by the teacher, and stressed the concept that the ends of rhyming words sound alike but the beginnings sound different (rhyme recognition). Next, the children practiced saying the five rhyme pairs in response to picture cues and clinician models (imitation). Finally, the clinicians and the children played a rhyme identification game.

Most rhyme identification games followed a simple sequence. Pictures representing one word from each of the rhyme pairs were placed faceup in front of the children. The clinicians held the other half of the pictures, which were introduced one by one. The children's job was to select the faceup picture that completed the rhyme pair, say the pair, then place the pictures in a pocket on the game board. For example, pictures representing the words *pox*, *toes*, *now*, *four*, and *spots* were placed in front of the children (book illustrations were used to picture the less concrete words such as *now*, and the children seemed to have no difficulty learning the picture-to-word matches). The clinicians showed the children a picture of a nose and said, "Which word rhymes with nose?" After one of the children selected the picture of toes, everyone said, "nose—toes" aloud. Then, one child put both pictures together into a pocket on the game board. This continued for the other four rhyme pairs.

During the second rhyming center of each week, the clinician reminded the children of the word pairs through an imitation activity. Then, the clinician and children played a rhyme judgment game in which the leader presented a picture of one target word paired with a picture of a word that did or did not rhyme. The children's task was to judge whether or not the two words rhymed. If they did not, the children were to provide the target word that correctly completed the rhyme.

Finally, the clinician and children played a rhyme production game. The clinician selected a rhyme pair and said, "Let's think of some other words that rhyme with *tie* and *high*. I know one: *tie*, *high*, *by*. Let's all say those." Children were encouraged to suggest other rhyming words. When they did, everyone said the three rhyming words aloud together. When they did not, the clinician provided the new rhyming word and the group said all three rhyming words together. This procedure was repeated for each of the five target rhyme pairs.

The same sequence of activities was repeated each week, except five new rhyme pairs were selected. After each 10 rhyming word pairs (two weeks), a new target rhyme book was selected and the new rhyming word pairs were selected from it.

Phonemic awareness intervention

Children in both classrooms worked on phoneme awareness during the spring semester. The purpose of the activities during that semester was to help the children acquire an awareness of sounds at the beginning and end of words. The authors developed a sequence of activities (see the box) based on the literature that was available on the development of phoneme awareness in children without specific language impairment. The target sounds were /b, d, g, m, n, s, f/. Two were presented each week.

Activities one through five in the box, which all focus on initial phonemes, were targeted during the first seven weeks of the semester. These activities were repeated for final sounds during weeks 8 through 10. The sound synthesis and analysis activities (7 and 8 in the box) were conducted during the final two weeks of the semester.

Intervention outcomes

Intervention resulted in significant improvement on measures of rhyming and phoneme awareness in the two groups of preschool children with

---

Sequence of Phoneme Awareness Activities

1. *Teach the initial sound–pictured word relationships.* The teacher and/or puppet tells children about the initial sounds in the eight target words.
2. *Initial position phoneme judgment and correction.* The child's task is to identify when words are said correctly or incorrectly. The child is asked to correct the teacher's or a puppet's incorrect production.
3. *Initial position sound matching.* Children pick pictures of words that begin with the sound that the teacher names.
4. *Initial sound identification.* The teacher selects a picture and the children tell the teacher what sound it starts with. Or children choose pictures and sort them into "sound bags."
5. *Generating words.* Children select untrained pictures of words that begin with target sounds, and think of words that begin with target sounds (no picture cues).
6. *Repeat the same four-step sequence with final position sounds.*
7. *Sound blending-synthesis.* The teacher says the component sounds (one at a time) in previously trained words. Children select the pictures. Then the teacher says the component sounds in previously untrained words. Children select the pictures.
8. *Sound analysis.* The teacher shows a picture of a previously trained word and says the word; children say the sounds. Then, the teacher shows a picture of a previously untrained word and says the word; children say the sounds.

language impairments who received training. The authors next asked whether this improvement could have been the result of general development rather than their training procedures. To answer this question, the authors compared their treatment groups with the older control group. The two treatment groups, whose rhyming abilities were significantly worse than those of the older control group at the beginning of the study, had caught up to the control subjects by the end of the study. These results indicated that the rhyming training was effective because one of the treatment groups was still a full year younger than the control subjects.

The findings for phoneme awareness were more dramatic. At the beginning of the study, children in all three groups performed poorly on the battery of phoneme awareness tasks. After training, the treatment groups (now aged, on average, 4;10 and 5;9) were significantly better than the six-year-old control subjects on these tasks. Clearly, the training resulted in changes beyond those that might have occurred if training had not been provided.

When the researchers explored the relationships between working memory and improvement in rhyming and phoneme awareness, they found low, negative correlations of −.33 and −.22, respectively. These low, negative correlations suggest that children with better phonological working memory at the outset were no more responsive to phonological awareness training than children with poorer phonological working memory. However, the authors do have evidence that training in phonological awareness had a positive impact on phonological coding abilities. Recall that nonword (but not real word) repetition abilities are believed to be a reasonably good indicator of phonological coding. The investigators found that real word repetition was essentially unchanged before and after training for both groups. However, the children who received training significantly improved their performance on nonword repetition tasks, implying that phonological awareness training did improve phonological aspects of working memory.

Finally, the researchers wondered whether improvements in phonological awareness affected the children's general preliteracy development. They correlated the children's improvement on rhyming and phoneme awareness with their posttreatment scores on a test of preliteracy development (the *Test of Early Reading Ability-2*; Reid, Hresko, & Hammill, 1989). The investigators found that phoneme awareness improvement, but not rhyming improvement, correlated significantly with the posttreatment measure of preliteracy development ($r = .51$). Recall that previous research has firmly established the relationship between phoneme awareness and early literacy development, particularly decoding abilities. The results of this study suggest that phoneme awareness training has educational implications even for preliteracy development.

•   •   •

Outcomes of an intervention study (Gillam & van Kleeck, in press) support the usefulness of phonological awareness training with children with language impairment. Intervention that focused on rhyming for one semester and then on phoneme awareness for a second semester resulted in improved phonological awareness abilities. Additionally, change in phonological awareness was significantly and positively related to a measure of early literacy ability. Working memory span at the beginning of the study did not predict responsiveness to the phonological awareness training, but phonological awareness training resulted in improvement in children's phonological coding abilities (an aspect of working memory) as measured by nonword repetition tasks.

Phonological awareness surely would not be the only focus the authors would advocate for late preschool and early school-age children with language disorders. Indeed, the children in the study participated in language intervention for other form, content, and use interactions at the same time they received the phonological awareness intervention. Although previous research has clearly shown that children with speech and language disorders are at high risk for reading disabilities, the authors recommend the inclusion of some form of phonological awareness training in intervention programs. Such training may fill an educational gap for all children (not just those with language impairments) who do not spontaneously acquire phonological awareness skills during the preschool years. These results suggest that such training should affect preliteracy development (and, by extension, early literacy development) as well as certain aspects of working memory.

REFERENCES

Adams, M.J. (1990). *Beginning to read: Thinking and learning about print.* Cambridge, MA: MIT Press.

Ball, E., & Blachman, B. (1991). Does phoneme awareness training in kindergarten make a difference in early word recognition and developmental spelling? *Reading Research Quarterly, 26*(1), 49–66.

Blachman, B. (1991). Early intervention for children's reading problems: Clinical applications of the research in phonological awareness. *Topics in Language Disorders, 12*(1), 51–65.

Bloom, L., & Lahey, M. (1978). *Language development and language disorders.* New York: Wiley.

Bradley, L., & Bryant, P. (1985). *Rhyme and reason in reading and spelling.* Ann Arbor: University of Michigan Press.

Brady, S. (1991). The role of working memory in reading disability. In S. Brady & D. Shankweiler (Eds.), *Phonological processes in literacy.* Hillsdale, NJ: Lawrence Erlbaum.

Byrne, B., & Fielding-Barnsley, R. (1991). Evaluation of a program to teach phonemic awareness to young children. *Journal of Educational Psychology, 83*, 451–455.

Cowan, N. (1995). *Attention and memory: An integrated framework.* New York: Oxford University Press.

Dollaghan, C.A. (1987). Fast mapping in normal and language-impaired children. *Journal of Speech and Hearing Disorders, 52*, 218–222.

Dowker, A. (1989). Rhyme and alliteration in poems elicited from young children. *Journal of Child Language, 16*, 181–202.

Ehri, L.C. (1992). Reconceptualizing the development of sight word reading and its relationship to recoding. In P.B. Gough, L.C. Ehri, & R. Treiman (Eds.), *Reading acquisition* (pp. 107–143). Hillsdale, NJ: Lawrence Erlbaum.

Ehri, L.C. (1994). Development of the ability to read words: Update. In R.B. Ruddell, M.R. Ruddell, & H. Singer (Eds.), *Theoretical models and processes of reading* (4th ed., pp. 323–358). Newark, DE: International Reading Association.

Fowler, A. (1991). How early phonological development might set the stage for phoneme awareness. In S. Brady & D. Shankweiler (Eds.), *Phonological processes in literacy.* Hillsdale, NJ: Lawrence Erlbaum.

Fox, B., & Routh, D. (1975). Analyzing spoken language into words, syllables, and phonemes. A developmental study. *Journal of Psycholinguistic Research, 4*, 331–342.

Fox, B., & Routh, D. (1984). Phonemic analysis and synthesis as word attack skills: Revisited. *Journal of Educational Psychology, 76*, 1059–1061.

Gathercole, S.E., & Baddeley, A.D. (1990). Phonological memory deficits in language disordered children: Is there a causal connection? *Journal of Memory and Language, 29*, 336–360.

Gathercole, S.E., & Baddeley, A.D. (1993). *Working memory and language.* Hillsdale, NJ: Lawrence Erlbaum.

Gillam, R., McFadden, T., & van Kleeck, A. (1995). Improving the narrative abilities of children with language disorders: Whole language and language skills approaches. In M. Fey, J. Windsor, & S. Warren (Eds.), *Language intervention: Preschool through the elementary years* (pp. 145–182). Baltimore: Brookes.

Gillam, R.B., & van Kleeck, A. (in press). A study of classroom-based phonological awareness training for preschoolers with speech and language disorders. *American Journal of Speech-Language Pathology.*

Jenkins, R., & Bowen, L. (1994). Facilitating development of preliterate children's phonological abilities. *Topics in Language Disorders, 12*(1), 26–39.

Lahey, M. (1988). *Language disorders and language development.* New York: Macmillan.

Lundberg, I., Frost, J., & Petersen, O. (1988). Effects of an extensive program for stimulating phonological awareness in preschool children. *Reading Research Quarterly, 23,* 363–384.

Maccarone, G., & Lewin, B. (1992). *Itchy, itchy chicken pox.* New York: Scholastic.

Maclean, M., Bryant, P., & Bradley, L. (1987). Rhymes, nursery rhymes, and reading in early childhood. *Merrill-Palmer Quarterly, 33*(3), 255–281.

Perfetti, C.A. (1992). The representation problem in reading acquisition. In P.B. Gough, L.C. Ehri, & R. Treiman (Eds.), *Reading acquisition* (pp. 145–174). Hillsdale, NJ: Lawrence Erlbaum.

Reid, D.K., Hresko, W., & Hammill, D. (1989). *Test of Early Reading Ability-2.* Austin, TX: PRO-ED.

Samuels, S.J. (1994). Word recognition. In R.B. Ruddell, M.R. Ruddell, & H. Singer (Eds.), *Theoretical models and processes of reading* (4th ed., pp. 359–380). Newark, DE: International Reading Association.

Torgesen, J.K., Morgan, S.T., & Davis, C. (1992). Effects of two types of phonological awareness training on word learning in kindergarten children. *Journal of Educational Psychology, 84,* 364–370.

Treiman, R. (1992). The role of intrasyllabic units in learning to read and spell. In P. Gough, L. Ehri, & R. Treiman (Eds.), *Reading acquisition* (pp. 65–106). Hillsdale, NJ: Lawrence Erlbaum.

van Kleeck, A. (1990). Emergent literacy: Learning about print before learning to read. *Topics in Language Disorders, 10*(2), 25–45.

van Kleeck, A. (1995). Emphasizing form and meaning separately in prereading and early reading instruction. *Topics in Language Disorders, 16*(1), 27–49.

Williams, J. (1980). Teaching decoding with an emphasis on phoneme analysis and phoneme blending. *Journal of Educational Psychology, 72,* 1–15.

6

Retraining Memory Strategies

Rick Parenté and Douglas Herrmann

Retraining a client's memory may take months, years, or a lifetime. Much of the therapist's success depends on factors that are difficult to control. Moreover, success in any stage of training cognitive function depends on success at the earlier stages of training. Rehearsal and attention/concentration are necessary precursors to memory strategy training. If the person cannot attend and concentrate reasonably well, memory strategies are virtually impossible to train (Eysenck, 1982). Likewise, if the person cannot maintain information in memory with rehearsal, then any type of strategy training is impossible (Gianutsos, 1991; Parenté & Anderson-Parenté, 1983; Schacter & Glisky, 1986). We assume, therefore, that the client's attention and sensory memory have already improved, and the client is now ready to relearn the skills of encoding, storage, and retrieval (Duffy, Walker, & Montague, 1972; Goldstein et al., 1988).

In this chapter, we focus on a variety of different memory strategies that the therapist can use to improve the client's ability to process information in working memory. These strategies are specifically designed to help the client store novel information in a form that can be easily retrieved (Atkinson & Wickens, 1971; Baddeley, 1986).

Source: Adapted from R. Parenté and D. Herrmann, "Retraining Memory Strategies," in *Retraining Cognition: Techniques and Applications*, pp. 105–114, © 1996, Aspen Publishers, Inc.

Top Lang Disord 1996;17(1):45–57
© 1996 Aspen Publishers, Inc.

Rehearsal is crucial for encoding because without rehearsal it would not be possible to maintain the information long enough to encode it. Likewise, encoding operations are crucial for efficient long-term memory functioning because without encoding, it is impossible to transform the information into a form that can be rapidly retrieved. Training to encode is perhaps the most important part of memory therapy (Hannon, de la Cruz-Schnedel, Cano, Moreira, & Nasuta, 1989; Harrell, Parenté, Bellingrath, & Lisicia, 1992; Kertesz, 1979).

Memory strategy training focuses on strategies and skills that transfer to the client's activities of daily living (Bellezza, 1981). Thus, it should be distinguished from other approaches that rely on mental exercise, such as stimulation therapy, which is designed to exercise the mind but not to teach the client strategies or skills. Although stimulation therapy may be useful for improving attention and concentration (Sarno, 1981; Wepman, 1951), it is questionable if it actually improves memory.

Simple mental exercise does not improve memory because no new learning takes place. This is because stimulation therapy approaches do not teach the client ways to process information more efficiently (Crosson & Buenning, 1984; Dansereau, 1985). They provide an environment for the client to practice remembering by using the same inefficient methods. The client can improve the speed of an inefficient system only to a certain level. However, unless he or she learns some new method of processing, the system will never function efficiently (Godfrey & Knight, 1988).

The basic value of stimulation therapy is the practice it affords. It may therefore be best used after the client has learned a number of different memory strategies because it provides an opportunity for practicing them. It can have the effect of priming the person for some type of activity (Payne & Wenger, 1992) or of warming up the memory system (Thune, 1950). However, if stimulation therapy forces the client to practice an already inefficient skill instead of acquiring new compensatory techniques, therapy may accomplish little in the way of improving memory.

Interest and motivation are critical to successful memory retraining. If a person with head injury is not interested in the training, this person will invariably perform at low levels. However, if a task is made interesting, performance will improve dramatically, and the person will attempt to use his or her newly learned skills in novel situations.

Incentives that affect learning and memory after head injury can be provided (Parenté & Herrmann, 1996). Without belaboring these points, it is clear that incentives can be provided in several ways. For example, the therapist can explain the task so that the client understands its relevance. The therapist can provide monetary incentives, making performance potentially lucrative or rewarding. Research with people who have not sustained a head injury has shown that monetary reward improves learning but not remembering. Apparently, a reward disposes people to try harder, but there is less effect on long-term memory. However, with survivors of head injury, monetary incentives dramatically improve memory and learning in a variety of memory tasks. The improvement from incentives has sometimes been as great as 400% to 600%.

THERAPY EXERCISES

We now present a variety of memory strategies, each suited for recall of certain types of information.

Training perceptual grouping of number series

We all must remember phone numbers, zip codes, extended zip codes, social security numbers, and other important numbers. Most people, however, recall number strings as sequences of individual digits. The average person can recall approximately seven digits correctly.

A typical phone number (seven digits) is not difficult to retain because it does not exceed most people's capacity. After head injury, however, the capacity of working memory is substantially reduced (roughly three to four units). Phone numbers, extended zip codes, or social security numbers may, therefore, overwhelm a person with head injury. Because the size of the digit string dramatically affects accuracy of recall, the trick to remembering digit strings is to group the digits into larger numbers. For example, many clients with head injury can recall three multidigit numbers (e.g., "324, 67, 31"), but they cannot recall seven individual digits (e.g., "3, 2, 4, 6, 7, 3, 1"). The therapist should therefore train clients to remember numbers in larger groupings or "chunks." We recommend the following step-by-step process.

Baseline

Present common number strings (e.g., zip codes, phone numbers) and ask the client to recall them. Determine the largest string the client can recall correctly.

Instruction

The first step is to train the client to pronounce groupings of digits as numbers. That is, the therapist should discourage the habit of remembering numbers as series of individual digits. This means that the therapist trains the client to remember two or three digits at a time by presenting them as individual digits but requiring the client to repeat them grouped into larger units. For example, the therapist may say "1, 2" and require the client to repeat the digits as "12." The therapist says "2, 3, 7" and requires the client to say "237." The therapist continues this type of training until the chunking translation is performed consistently and automatically.

Although it is always possible to train clients to use the strategy, it is more difficult to ensure that they learn to use it automatically. It is therefore unreasonable to expect that simply demonstrating the strategy is sufficient to get the client to use it. Most clients will require extensive practice using the strategy. Some clients may learn to do the perceptual grouping operation in 50 trials. Others take hundreds before the technique becomes second nature. The important point is that the client must learn to use the strategy automatically.

The second step is to increase the number of digits and have the client recall multiple higher-order groupings. For example, say "3, 4, 6, 8" and require "34, 68" as a response. The goal at this stage is to get the person to recall numbers the size of a zip code, using the grouping strategy. The therapist teaches the client to recall a zip code as a three-digit number and a two-digit number. For example, if the therapist says "2, 6, 8, 5, 4," the client should respond, "268, 54" or "26, 854."

The therapist should assign homework that requires the client to read lists of digit strings and practice the groupings as words. For example, create lists of digit strings such as "3, 4, 5, 6, 3" and have the client practice grouping the various strings (e.g., "345, 63").

Generalization

Once the client groups digits automatically, the therapist can continue training with commonly used numbers such as phone numbers, social security numbers, and extended zip codes. The client should learn to group a phone number as a three-digit number followed by two, two-digit numbers. The client can also learn to remember a social security number as a three-digit number followed by three groups of two digits. This same grouping structure works well for extended zip codes. Clients can learn to recall extended phone numbers (with area code) as two three-digit numbers (area code and prefix) followed by two, two-digit numbers.

Persons with head injury who internalize this strategy to the point at which they use it automatically do not have any problem remembering numbers. Once again, the difficulty is getting them to use it automatically. To convince them that the strategy is effective, the therapist should test their multidigit, multinumber memory at the beginning of training. She or he can then test it again at the end to demonstrate the improvement when using the strategy.

One test procedure involves finding a phone number in the phone directory and asking the client to call the information operator and get the number for that person. The client then repeats the number to the therapist in grouped form, and the therapist validates it from the directory.

Training organization

Baseline

Once again, the first step in training any memory skill is to collect baseline data. However, there are so many semantic organizational procedures that it is difficult to specify one as most indicative of the client's skill level. We suggest using a list-learning procedure in which the items can be grouped into several categories (e.g., fruits, vegetables). After reading the list, the client recalls the words and the therapist determines if the words are remembered according to the various groupings. The critical measure here is whether the words are semantically grouped at recall. Usually they are not because the ability to perceive semantic organization is disrupted.

Instruction

The therapist types word lists of various lengths onto 3-by-5 cards and trains the client to sort the cards into the various categorical piles. For example, the client may place all vegetable items in one pile and all dairy products in another.

The first step trains recognition of the hierarchical organization of the list. The client later uses the organizational structure as a retrieval cue. The therapist trains the client to recognize the various categories before attempting to recall the individual elements. The therapist asks the client to recall not the individual items on the list but the structural categories (e.g., vegetables, household materials, meats). This procedure forces recognition of the categories, which will later serve as a cuing aid. The number of categories should never exceed the client's working memory capacity (usually three to five units).

In the second step, the client continues with the sorting and recall procedure but recalls as well the specific words after the category. Once the client has learned the categories, recall of the actual items is relatively easy. Most clients are amazed that after they learn the categories, the words fall into place automatically.

The session should always begin by the therapist's presenting a body of seemingly disorganized information and having the client try to remember it using whatever strategies he or she may choose. Word lists are easy to construct. Other simple materials such as a random assortment of household or office items also work well. The therapist simply places 10 to 15 items on the tabletop and asks the client to remember what is there. The person may not be able to recall more than four or five items without the organization strategy, even after repeated study and test. But after training to focus on the organization rather than the elements, most clients easily recall 12 items in five or six study/test sessions, a 100% savings. Showing clients how much they improve their recall with this procedure is the most important portion of the therapy. Once clients see that it works, they are more likely to use it outside of the therapy context.

The therapist should provide clients with at least 50 words and instructions to make up lists of at least 10 words at a time. They can then practice the sequence of steps on their own and demonstrate their skill during later therapy sessions.

When clients are unable to use semantic categories to improve their recall, the therapist should try other organizational categories that are more concrete, such as color categories, acoustic similarities among the words, formal similarity (e.g., coat, boat), or spatial similarity (e.g., in the same room). Ideally, any set of training materials (words, objects, shapes) should have some relevance to the person's daily life, and the training should focus on whatever organizational strategy produces the highest levels of recall.

Generalization

The therapist should continue training with practical activities to determine if the client can generalize the strategy. We recommend the following exercises:

- Family members can provide a simple household task they would like the client to do (e.g., wash the car). The client can then do the task by categorizing the materials needed and the correct sequence of steps to perform the task (e.g., "What is necessary in order to wash the family car? Cleaning materials, washing devices, and so forth"). After the person has recalled the categories, he or she should try to recall the materials individually.
- Alphabetizing names is a simple and useful activity. Ideally, these should be the names of friends or acquaintances so that clients can simultaneously relearn their social environment. Eventually, clients should sort by zip code, north-south east-west portions of their locale, street names, and so forth.
- The family can provide 20 to 30 household items and have the client reorganize them into appropriate categories (e.g., living room, eating utensils, laundry items).
- The client can be asked to read a few paragraphs of text and write an outline from memory. The client should reread the text until he or she can correctly outline the materials.

Training mediation

Self-questioning

Mediation strategies involve training clients to establish an association between the new thing they are trying to learn and something familiar. The therapist's goal is to get clients always to ask a certain set of questions about the new thing. These include "What does it look like? What does it sound like? What does it smell like? What does it taste like? What does it mean the same thing as? What groups does it belong to? Who is it commonly associated with?" Such questions simply focus attention on the formal, meaningful, spatial, or other similarity of the to-be-remembered person or event and its association to something the client already knows.

The questions begin with "Who? What? When? Where? How? Why?" Thus, when making a new acquaintance, the client might ask, "Whom does the person look like? What does the person's name sound like? To what nationality does the person seem to belong? What type of perfume or cologne is the person wearing? Where did I meet the person? What were the distinct characteristics of the person's face or body? When (what time) did I meet the person? How did the meeting take place? Why was I introduced?" When the client tries to recall the person later, he or she again tries to answer the same questions. The technique works because it allows the client to establish multiple retrieval routes to the same core memory. When he or she is trying to recall the event later, one or more of the retrieval routes is likely to reproduce the memory.

Sentence mnemonics

Other techniques of mediation, called *mnemonics*, are also quite effective with certain clients. *Sentence mnemonics* are sentences that cue our memories for lists of words or instructions (Bower & Winzenz, 1970; Herrmann, Geissler, & Atkinson, 1973). For example, recalling the words *baby, cow, glass, tree,* and *steel* is considerably easier if a client learns to create a sentence such as "The baby cow eats steel near the glass tree." Clearly, this sentence is bizarre. However, it has the effect of integrating the previously unrelated words into an easily rehearsed unit.

Baseline

Have the client freely recall a list of unrelated words. The initial level of recall is the baseline.

Instruction

First, using a different set of words, teach the client to form a bizarre sentence that relates the words. Record how many trials it takes the client to say the sentence that includes all the words. After the client can say the entire sentence from memory, point out that the sentence also contained the entire list of words. This may be obvious to some clients, but it will not be for most. In any case, the exercise will demonstrate the utility of the technique.

Next, teach the client to use the sentence to recall the words alone—that is, to use the sentence as a mediator. Specifically, the client should speak the sentence subvocally and use the sentence to recall the words.

Last, illustrate improvement of recall using the sentence mnemonic strategy with another set of words. Clients often complain that bizarre sentences are meaningless and irrelevant. Actually, there is no good reason for the sentence to be bizarre. Any sentence will work as long as it integrates the words.

Generalization

After considerable training, clients will begin to produce sentence mnemonics on their own to deal with things they must remember in everyday life. This is the primary goal of the therapy.

Word mnemonics

Simple words can be especially useful mnemonics. One problem-solving technique can be summarized by the SOLVE mnemonic: (S)pecify the problem—define it; (O)ptions—what are they? (L)isten to advice from others; (V)ary the solution; (E)valuate the effect of the solution—did it really solve the problem?

Another word mnemonic is designed to help clients control their anger. It includes the two words *anger* and *calm*. The ANGER sequence is as follows: (A)nticipate the signs of anger; (N)ever act in anger; (G)o through the CALM sequence; (E)valuate the situation; (R)eview how you coped. The CALM sequence is as follows: (C)all someone for help; (A)llow yourself to emote; (L)eave the situation; (M)ove about. This is a psychosocial mnemonic that teaches the person to recognize what makes him or her angry as well as the physical signs of anger (e.g., increased body temperature, clenched fist). The client learns never to take any action while angry—that is, before going through the CALM sequence.

The first step in the CALM sequence is to call someone for help and allow the emotion to escape in a sympathetic environment. The client should also make every effort to leave the situation that is causing the anger and to move about in order to dissipate the anger. Once the client has gone through the CALM sequence, then he or she can return to the E portion of the anger mnemonic. At this point, the client is in a better position to evaluate the situation rationally and to determine what it was that caused the anger. Finally, the client learns to review what facilitated coping with the anger and to write it down for later review.

Another word mnemonic, LISTEN, is designed to teach the client effective listening skills: (L)ook at the person who is talking—maintain eye contact; (I)nterest yourself in the topic; (S)peak less than half the time; (T)ry not to interrupt or change the topic; (E)valuate what is said—don't blindly accept it; (N)otice facial expressions and body positions. We have found that rehearsing these points while the client is listening can dramatically improve attention and memory for conversations.

Generalization

Once the client understands the concept of word mnemonics, it is feasible to work with him or her to develop individual mnemonics that may be uniquely helpful. We will typically ask clients to discuss their biggest memory problems to determine if a mnemonic can help. For example, one client was in mechanics training and could not recall all of the things he was supposed to check on a car that came into the shop. He could not use a checklist because it would get greasy and unreadable. We developed the LITE BRACE mnemonic and worked with the client until he had memorized it: (L)ook and listen, (I)gnition, (T)ransmission, (E)xhaust, (B)rakes, (R)ear end, (A)ir conditioning, (C)oolant, (E)lectrical. The advantage of this mnemonic for the client was that it solved a major problem. He was therefore quite motivated to learn it and to use it in his training.

Another client sustained a severe right hemisphere injury. Her speech was disinhibited, and there were several complaints that she would go off on tangents and lose the focus of her points in conversation. We therefore developed the BOMS mnemonic for her to remind her of how to explain her points clearly and efficiently: (B)ottom line, (O)mit the details, (M)odulate your voice for emphasis, (S)ummarize your point at the end.

Rhyming mnemonics

Rhymes are especially effective for training long-term retention of semantic information and procedures. For example, many of us learned the rhyme for remembering the number of days in each month of the year: "Thirty days hath September, April, June, and November. All the rest have 31 except the second month alone, to which we 28 assign, till leap year gives it 29." Rhymes are difficult to create but have lasting effects on memory.

Instruction

First, provide the client with several rhymes that illustrate the concept of rhyming mnemonics. For example, rhymes that most of us learn in grade school, such as "*i* before *e* except after *c*" or "30 days hath September," are appropriate. These also provide the client with valuable tools to cue specific recall that can be used for a lifetime.

Once the client has mastered these rhymes, original rhymes can be developed. Therapy may never progress beyond the point at which the therapist develops rhymes that the client memorizes. Nevertheless, time spent developing useful rhymes is time well spent. The more the client invests in the process, the more relevance the rhymes will have. Ideally, the client will come to develop personal rhymes with the therapist's assistance at first. For example, one client had difficulty remembering to ask "who, what, when, where, why, and how" in order to organize novel information.

He developed, with the therapist, the following rhyme to assist his use of the strategy: "To remember in the here and now, ask who, what, when, where, why, and how. To remember it again, ask who, what, where, how, why, and when."

Last, have the client try related tasks that demonstrate mastery of the rhyme. For example, after memorizing the rhyme "*i* before *e* except after *c* and for sounds like *eigh,* as in *neighbor* or *weigh,*" the client should attempt to spell the words (e.g., *conceive* versus *thief*), and after memorizing "30 days hath September," the client should attempt to tell how many days there are in the various months.

Generalization

Have the family members select everyday behaviors that the client can integrate into a rhyme. For example, lists of things to do before leaving the house are always useful. Rules for operating household appliances have obvious practical value. One client had difficulty remembering to lock her door and turn out lights before going to bed. She lived in the inner city in a neighborhood where there were several break-ins. Her neighbor mentioned that he could see into her apartment window while she was undressing. Her family and she created this rhyme: "Lock the door—turn out the lights. Draw the blinds—block out the sights."

Training mental imagery

The visual analogue to the strategies described thus far is mental imagery. Training imagery may not work well with low-functioning clients or those with residual right hemisphere lesions. It does work well with those who have made greater gains in recovery. Training imagery is easiest when the task is to recall concrete items. It does not work well for abstractions. For example, it is easy to remember a visual scene such as a baseball player hitting a home run. However, it may be impossible to imagine symbolic concepts such as truth, justice, or the American way. Imagery is most effective when the parts of the image actively interact (Higbee, 1988; McDaniel & Pressley, 1987; Richardson, 1992).

Baseline

Collect baseline data on a memory task such as memorizing a word list.

Instruction

First, demonstrate the concept of a mental image. With eyes closed, the client conjures up the image of his or her mother's face. Alternatively, he or she can draw a map of a familiar place. Either of these activities demonstrates the concept of a mental image.

Then demonstrate the power of a mental image. For example, have the client recall a list of 12 words. We typically read the following list and ask the client to recall the words after hearing the list: "Bowl, Passion, Fruit, Judge, Dawn, Bee, Plane, County, Choice, Seed, Wool, and Meal." The therapist reads the list again and the client attempts a second recall. The process continues for several trials. Typically, the client will not recall the words even after several study and test trials.

The therapist then instructs the client to use mental imagery. The client is asked to close his or her eyes and, while the therapist reads another word list, to try to form a mental image of the words in his or her mind. For example, we usually use the following list image: "Think of a DOG chasing a CAT up a TREE. Behind the tree is a ROAD. On the road is a CADILLAC. ELVIS is driving the Cadillac. Behind the road is the SKY. In the sky is a full MOON. In front of the moon is a WITCH. The witch is riding a BROOM. Beneath the witch is a STAR. Behind the star is the ENTERPRISE."

After the client hears the image, he or she attempts recall of the word lists using the mental image to mediate recall. Most clients can recall the entire word list in two trials, whereas they cannot recall the first word list even after six or more study and test trials. This demonstration illustrates the power of mental imagery.

Generalization

Ask the client to close his or her eyes and imagine a familiar map such as that of the United States. Ask questions such as "What direction would you travel if you went from Chicago to Dallas?" Or ask the client to close his or her eyes, then place a familiar object in the client's hands (e.g., a key). Instruct the client to form a mental image of what it looks like. Then verbally describe it in detail. Repeat this technique with a second and a third object. Eventually give the person an object that is similar or identical to the first. Ask the client to identify it as same or different. If different, ask, "Why is it different?" Begin with five object pairs. For example, use two keys, two coins, pencil and pen, two types of paper clips, and two erasers; then gradually expand the set to 10 items. Show the client pictures of unfamiliar faces and ask for a verbal description or a sketch of each face after removing the picture from view. Have the client, with eyes closed, trace familiar objects with the index finger (e.g., circle, square, triangle). Ask the client to say what the object is. Gradually make the shapes more complex. Give the client verbal directions how to get somewhere, then have the client draw the corresponding map.

Imagery may be quite difficult for most persons with head injury to learn. Nevertheless, it is a powerful memory aid and may be quite useful. In our experience, imagery training is less useful for remembering things like lists but more useful when viewed as part of other, more functional memory tasks such as name-face association or recall of text materials. It is therefore necessary to tell the client that he or she will use imagery in a variety of memory strategies and to point out when it is used. Usually, clients did not knowingly use imagery before their injury. Therefore, they may have no clear idea of what the term *mental image* means. Extensive demonstration of the concept and its power may be necessary before the clients can use the strategy effectively. The therapist should gradually make the images more complex.

Training associative memory

Survivors of head injury frequently have difficulty forming associations. For example, they may have a hard time recalling names after an initial introduction or learning and associating a phone number with a newly acquired friend. Lack of attention and poor rehearsal are the biggest reasons that they cannot form associations easily. For example, they may avoid eye contact when meeting new people. They seldom realize how many rehearsals are necessary before the information will stick in memory. As with the other memory tasks, retraining associative learning is a sequential process.

It is usually best to start with relatively simple associations and gradually progress to the more difficult ones. Again, we recommend constructing training materials that are similar to those the client will encounter in everyday life.

Baseline

Present the client with word-picture associations to learn. For example, the therapist could take photographs of everyone the client sees in the rehabilitation center or outpatient clinic and write the appropriate name on the back of each picture. The therapist would then present these pictures one at a time and ask the client to recall the names. The therapist should then record the number of study and test trials necessary to associate the names correctly.

Instruction

Initiate the training by providing the client with the letter mnemonic NAME: (N)otice the person—maintain eye contact; (A)sk the person to spell and pronounce his or her name; (M)ention the name in conversation; (E)xaggerate some facial feature.

Rehearsal of the names and faces is a psychosocial skill that trains the client to do whatever is necessary to elicit enough rehearsal of the name. For example, pretending that he or she did not hear the name or asking the person to spell it is useful for getting the person to say the name again. The client must hear the name several times in order to ensure adequate rehearsal.

Provide feedback about the number of rehearsal trials necessary before the client can learn the name-face association. From that point on, require that many rehearsals before the client attempts recall.

If snapshots are not available, construct flash cards with pictures selected from magazines. Each card should display a person's face with no name. Initially, ask the client to make up names that would fit the faces. This forces attention to facial features that will cue the name.

Next, show pictures of faces and ask the client to sketch cartoons of the faces, exaggerating some facial feature. This activity promotes effective scanning and attention to salient facial cues. The technique is similar to that used by political cartoonists who exaggerate one facial feature (e.g., Richard Nixon's nose, Jimmy Carter's teeth). The cartoon creates an unforgettable image of the person in the public eye. Likewise, drawing a cartoon image of a new acquaintance on the back of a business card or next to his or her phone number in an address book can aid recall of the person later on.

Now have the client practice the introduction and rehearsal process with another person and videotape the encounter. Afterward, play the tape and ask which aspects of the NAME process the client did well and which ones need work.

The client should go through the sequence of steps whenever he or she is introduced to someone. Eventually, the sequence becomes second nature, and the client's memory for names and faces improves noticeably.

Generalization

The best evidence that clients have learned to associate names and faces is to observe whether they use the strategies just outlined spontaneously when they are introduced to new people. The therapy should continue until clients implement the techniques without prompting.

•   •   •

This chapter provides step-by-step instructions for training various memory encoding strategies. It emphasizes only strategies that are simple and have proven effective. Perceptual grouping of number strings into chunks typically facilitates rehearsal and memory of number strings. Training rhymes can improve memory for specific sets of activities. Training mental organization will improve the client's ability to formulate retrieval cues (Ellis & Hunt, 1993).

For all of these strategies, training involves collecting baseline data, providing instruction, determining if instruction improves retention, and, if so, continuing training. It is also necessary to determine if the training generalizes to real-world activities.

The eventual goal of therapy is to train the client to use the strategies spontaneously. Long-term episodic retention involves continued training with the encoding skills outlined above. The client will probably always demonstrate some impairment of long-term retention for episodic information. However, these mnemonic strategies may help clients compensate for their memory difficulties.

Initially, the client may feel that mnemonics are too difficult to use or they require too much cognitive effort. Eventually, however, the person will realize that it is easier to remember and use the devices than it is not to use them. But this type of training requires patience, long-term persistence, and application in a real-world context. Generalization of the strategies may not occur for several months, or perhaps a year or more. It is, therefore, never sufficient simply to demonstrate the procedures and assume that the client will spontaneously apply them from that point on.

Training memory is an art. It requires patience and time. Many of the strategies outlined above may not work with a particular client. Therefore, one of the therapist's functions is to assess the various strategies until one or more can be isolated that are uniquely suited to a particular client. If the client learns even one strategy and utilizes it spontaneously, the time taken to learn it was well spent.

REFERENCES

Atkinson, R.C., & Wickens, T.D. (1971). Human memory and the concept of reinforcement. In R. Glaser (Ed.), *The nature of reinforcement*. London: Academic Press.

Baddeley, A.D. (1986). *Working memory*. New York: Basic Books.

Bellezza, F.S. (1981). Mnemonic devices: Classification, characteristics, and criteria. *Review of Education Research, 51*, 247–275.

Bower, G.H., & Winzenz, D. (1970). Comparison of associative learning strategies. *Psychonomic Science, 20*, 119–120.

Crosson, B., & Buenning, W. (1984). An individualized memory retraining program after closed-head injury: A single-case study. *Journal of Clinical Neuropsychology, 6*, 287–301.

Dansereau, D.F. (1985). Learning strategy research. In J.W. Segal, S.F. Chipman, & R. Glasser (Eds.), *Thinking and learning skills* (Vol. 1). Hillsdale, NJ: Lawrence Erlbaum.

Duffy, T.M., Walker, C., & Montague, W.E. (1972). Sentence mnemonics and the role of verb-class in paired-associate learning. *Psychological Reports, 31*, 583–589.

Ellis, H.C., & Hunt, R.R. (1993). *Fundamentals of cognitive psychology*. Madison, WI: W.C. Brown and Benchmark.

Eysenck, M.W. (1982). *Attention and arousal: Cognition and performance*. Berlin: Academic Press.

Gianutsos, R. (1991). Cognitive rehabilitation: A neuropsychological specialty comes of age. *Brain Injury, 5*, 353–368.

Godfrey, H., & Knight, R. (1988). Memory training and behavioral rehabilitation of a severely head-injured adult. *Archives of Physical Medicine Rehabilitation, 69*, 458–460.

Goldstein, G., McCue, M., Turner, S., Spanier, E., Malec, E., & Shelly, C. (1988). An efficacy study of memory training for patients with closed-head injury. *Clinical Neuropsychologist, 2*, 252–259.

Hannon, R., de la Cruz-Schnedel, D., Cano, T., Moreira, K., & Nasuta, R. (1989). Memory retraining with adult male alcoholics. *Archives of Clinical Neuropsychology, 4*, 227–232.

Harrell, M., Parenté, R., Bellingrath, E.G., & Lisicia, K.A. (1992). *Cognitive rehabilitation of memory: A practical guide*. Gaithersburg, MD: Aspen.

Herrmann, D.J., Geissler, F.V., & Atkinson, R.C. (1973). The serial position function for lists learned by a narrative-story mnemonic. *Bulletin of the Psychonomic Society, 2,* 377–378.

Higbee, K.L. (1988). *Your memory* (2nd ed.). Englewood Cliffs, NJ: Prentice Hall.

Kertesz, A. (1979). *Aphasia and associated disorders: Taxonomy, localization, and recovery*. New York: Grune & Stratton.

McDaniel, M.A., & Pressley, M. (1987). *Imagery and related mnemonic processes: Theories, individual differences and applications*. New York: Springer-Verlag.

Parenté, F.J., & Anderson-Parenté, J.K. (1983). Techniques for improving cognitive rehabilitation: Teaching organization and encoding skills. *Journal of Cognitive Rehabilitation, 1*(4), 20–23.

Parenté, R., & Herrmann, D. (1996). *Retraining cognition: Techniques and applications*. Gaithersburg, MD: Aspen.

Payne, D., & Wenger, M.J. (1992). Memory improvement and practice. In D. Herrmann, H. Weingartner, A. Searleman, & C. McEvoy (Eds.), *Memory improvement: Implications for memory theory* (pp. 187–209). New York: Springer-Verlag.

Richardson, J.T.E. (1992). Imagery mnemonics and memory remediation. *Neurology, 42,* 283–286.

Sarno, M.T. (1981). Recovery and rehabilitation in aphasia. In M.T. Sarno (Ed.), *Acquired aphasia*. New York: Academic Press.

Schacter, D.L., & Glisky, E.L. (1986). Memory remediation: Restoration, alleviation, and the acquisition of domain-specific knowledge. In B. Uzzell & Y. Gross (Eds.), *Clinical neuropsychology of intervention* (pp. 257–282). New York: Martinus Nijhoff.

Thune, L.E. (1950). The effect of different types of preliminary activities on subsequent learning of paired-associate material. *Journal of Experimental Psychology, 40,* 423–438.

Wepman, J.M. (1951). *Recovery from aphasia*. New York: Ronald.

PART II

Long-Term Memory and Language Impairment

"Oh, I Remember Now!": Facilitating Children's Long-Term Memory for Events

Judith A. Hudson and Ronald B. Gillam

Jennifer, age 8, was participating in a study on memory. During one of her sessions, the examiner, who knew Jennifer had been taking horseback-riding lessons for about three months, asked her to tell him how to saddle a horse. She responded,

> You brush him. And then you put the saddle on. And then you put the girth on. And then you put the bridle on. And then you get on.

When Jennifer met with the examiner a few days later, he asked her to explain how to saddle a horse again. This time, however, he handed Jennifer a toy horse with a saddle and a bridle. Holding the horse in her hand, Jennifer responded,

> Well, first you brush it. And then you have to pick a hoof. And you have to pick all the hoofs. And then you brush him all down his body and everything. And then you have to brush his tail. And you brush it to make it not get so tangly, and his mane. And then you have to put on a saddle pad. And then, um, you usually have to tighten the girth. And it goes kind of like a seat belt. You have to tighten it, but usually they'll blow up their stomach because they don't want it too tight.

Preparation of this article was supported, in part, by a grant from the National Institute on Deafness and Other Communication Disorders to the second author.

Top Lang Disord 1997;18(1):1–15

And then you have to put on the bridle. Then, go back and check the girth again. And then you should, um, get on.

Jennifer's parents were certain that she knew even more about saddling a horse than what she had described in the second session. They observed Jennifer and took notes as she saddled her horse just before a riding lesson. Jennifer successfully completed a 21-step process without any suggestions from her instructor. Clearly, Jennifer knew far more about saddling a horse than she could tell, even while viewing a prop.

What do Jennifer's retellings and actions tell us about her language and memory abilities? Why was she able to recall so much more information during the second session than she was during the first session? Why was her actual performance of the steps involved in saddling a horse so much more complex than her telling?

Recent research has produced a wealth of data on what children remember over long periods of time. Until 1985, the study of children's long-term memory was dominated by research on children's recall in directed memory tasks that took place in laboratory contexts. Results indicated that preschool children were unable to use deliberate memory strategies and, consequently, showed little evidence of long-term recall. In the last decade, however, researchers have generally acknowledged that research on memory strategies has misrepresented young children's memory abilities, and research has increasingly focused on children's memory for real-world events (Schneider & Bjorklund, in press). In contrast to their poor performance on directed memory tasks, young children can accurately remember information from real-world events over very long periods of time. This type of memory is acquired implicitly by participating in real-world events, it is retrieved without conscious awareness, and it can include both declarative (facts acquired through learning) and procedural (actions and skills) memory.

FACTORS THAT INFLUENCE LONG-TERM EVENT MEMORY

A consistent finding across numerous studies is that when asked to provide a verbal account of a past event, preschool children's reports are typically less complete than those of older children (e.g., Baker-Ward, Gordon, Ornstein, Larus, & Clubb, 1993; Fivush, Haden, & Adam, 1995; Hudson, 1990a). There are several variables that could account for these developmental differences. One possibility is that younger children initially encode less information about events and, therefore, produce less information at time of recall. An alternative possibility is that developmental differences are a result of memory changes that affect storage. There may be developmental differences in the rate of memory decay or in the degree to which event information is altered in memory. It is also possible that younger children have more difficulty with the retrieval process. They may be less able to use cues in the recall context, or they may have difficulty constructing an internal search. Finally, younger children may simply lack the verbal skills to report all that they can remember.

Of course, these processes are not independent. How an event is encoded will affect the kinds of cues that are needed for retrieval. Changes in the way information is stored will affect how readily the information can later be retrieved. Additionally, children's verbal ability will certainly influence both encoding and retrieval processes. Nevertheless, an encoding-storage-retrieval-reporting framework is useful for considering the role of developmental differences in different phases of recall and may help to identify aspects of recall that are susceptible to effects of language delay.

DEVELOPMENTAL DIFFERENCES IN ENCODING

Research from laboratory studies indicates that older children employ more deliberate encoding strategies in directed memory tasks (Kail, 1989). Consequently, older children form stronger memory traces for stimulus materials than do younger children (Brainerd, Reyna, Howe, & Kingma, 1990). Strong memory traces fade more slowly than weak memory traces, resulting in better long-term retention for older children. Nelson (1994) has proposed that very young children (under three years of age) may be slower to consolidate event memories as compared with older children, and their memories may be more vulnerable to disruption.

Age differences in encoding have also been attributed to developmental differences in children's knowledge bases. For example, Pillemer, Picariello, and Pruett (1994) conducted a longitudinal investigation of preschool children's memory for a fire drill. They found that seven years after the event, children who were four-and-a-half years of age at the time of the fire drill recalled significantly more information than children who were three-and-a-half years old. Older children's memory reports were more coherent and showed a clearer understanding of the causes of the event and the sequence of activities, suggesting that their initial encoding of the event was more complete than that of the younger children.

As the Pillemer et al. study indicates, age differences in encoding are largely attributed to age differences in event knowledge that provide older children with a more coherent framework for understanding novel events. Despite the fact that older children generally have more knowledge about many events than do younger children, knowledge-base effects have been found to be independent of age. For example, children with more prior knowledge about physical examinations remember more about a visit to the pediatrician because their prior knowledge can influence the encoding, storage, and interpretation of the experience (Baker-Ward et al., 1993; Ornstein, Gordon, & Larus, 1992). In a study of children's memory for an invasive medical procedure (the voiding cystourethrogram [VCUG]), Goodman, Quas, Batterman-Faunce, Riddlesberger, and Kuhn (1994) showed that children who were provided with more information about the procedure beforehand recalled more information than children who were given less information.

These findings are consistent with research on how script knowledge affects children's event memory. *Script knowledge* or *general event knowledge* refers to schematically organized knowledge about the expected sequence of actions in familiar events. Script knowledge can provide an organized framework to guide encoding and retrieval of memories of specific events (see Hudson, 1993b, and Naremore, Chapter 8, for reviews).

However, script knowledge can also make it difficult to distinguish specific episodes of routine events from general event representations. Younger children (ages three to four) are generally less able than older children (ages five to seven) to distinguish specific episodes from general script knowledge (Farrar & Goodman, 1990; Hudson, 1993b).

Degree of participation in an event has also been found to affect children's encoding. When an event is personally experienced, it is likely that a stronger memory trace will be found than if an event is merely observed (Ornstein, Larus, & Clubb, 1991). Several lines of investigation support this claim. Children generally recall more information from events that they experience directly than events that they observe or learn about through stories (Baker-Ward, Hess, & Flannagan, 1990; Foley & Johnson, 1985; Rudy & Goodman, 1991).

Finally, the discussion of an event during encoding can also affect children's ability to recall that event at a later time. Tessler and Nelson

(1994) studied three- and four-year-old children's memory for a visit to a museum with their mothers. Children recalled more information about objects seen on the trip if they had been mentioned during the trip than if they had been seen but not mentioned. Three-year-olds, in particular, were unable to verbally recall any object that had not been mentioned during the original trip. However, children were able to recognize objects that were seen but not talked about, suggesting that young children are able to retain in memory information that is not verbally accessible.

Although variables affecting encoding have been shown to operate independently of age differences in children's use of strategies, their knowledge base, the degree to which they are able to distinguish episodes from generic scripts, and the degree to which they are able to verbally participate in an event may all contribute to developmental differences in long-term recall. Howe and O'Sullivan (1997) argue that it is often difficult to fully evaluate the role of storage and retrieval processes in long-term retention because so few memory studies can rule out initial developmental differences in encoding.

DEVELOPMENTAL DIFFERENCES IN STORAGE

There are several ways in which memories may be altered in storage. First, over longer time delays, memories of specific episodes become more generic and script-like as they become blended with general event knowledge. Children tend to confuse details from multiple similar experiences such as repeated play events (Farrar & Goodman, 1990), creative movement workshops (Hudson, 1990b), birthday parties (Hudson & Nelson, 1986), and medical examinations (Ornstein, Shapiro, Clubb, Follner, & Baker-Ward, 1996). Younger children appear to be more influenced by script knowledge than older children. They recall more script-consistent than script-inconsistent information over longer time delays (Shapiro, Clubb, & Ornstein, 1995) and generate more confusion and script-related intrusions in recall (Farrar & Goodman, 1990).

Time also affects changes in memories in that central information is retained longer than peripheral details (Howe & Brainerd, 1989; Howe, O'Sullivan, & Marche, 1992). A study of one-and-a-half to five-year-old children's memory for traumatic experiences (visits to a hospital emergency department) over a six-month interval found that, over time, children continued to report central information but excluded many details that had been present in their reports a few days following treatment (Howe, Courage, & Peterson, 1995). In a longitudinal study of kindergarten children's memory for a museum trip, Hudson and Fivush (1991) found that six years after the trip, children were more likely to recall the most salient features of the trip and were less likely to remember peripheral information, such as walking to the museum, even when they were provided with photograph cues of the less salient actions.

Changes in children's knowledge base over time can also contribute to changes in their memory reports. In the study of children's memory for a trip to a museum of archaeology mentioned above (Hudson & Fivush, 1991), children tended to add details in their later memory reports that were not present in the accounts they gave immediately after the trip. For example, as kindergartners, they were delighted to find real artifacts, but as sixth-graders, they reported that the artifacts had been "planted" in the sandbox. Thus, when children's world knowledge changes, they may reconstruct memories of earlier experiences in ways that are consistent with their new understandings (Howe & Brainerd, 1989; Myles-Worsley, Cromer, & Dodd, 1986).

Intervening similar experiences can also alter memories. Events that were originally experienced as novel and distinctive, after repeated experiences, become less distinctive and less distinguishable from a generic script. A follow-up investigation of children's memory for emergency department visits discussed above showed that children who experienced subsequent emergency department visits tended to confuse information from separate episodes (Howe, 1995).

Although reexperiencing an event makes it more difficult to distinguish between particular episodes, overall event memory is strengthened by reenactment. Fivush and Hamond (1989) found that 24- and 28-month-old children who reenacted several three-step action sequences two weeks after their initial training recalled more actions after three months than children who were not given the chance to reenact the actions. Hudson and Sheffield (in press) found that 18-month-olds recalled more action sequences over a delay of two to eight months if they had reenacted the actions during the delay.

Reexperiencing part of an event can also refresh children's event recall through the process of reinstatement (Campbell & Jaynes, 1966). Reinstatement is distinguished from reenactment in that children are not given the opportunity to reproduce an event in its entirety. Rather, they are passively exposed to partial information about a past event. Howe, Courage, and Bryant-Brown (1992) investigated reinstatement of preschool children's memories using a hiding task. Two- and three-year-old children were shown the hiding places of 16 toys located in a playroom. One week later, half of the children returned to the room and were shown the toys but not the locations. In recall testing three weeks later, children who had participated in the reinstatement session recalled more locations than children who received no reinstatement. Sheffield and Hudson (1994) found that 14- and 18-month-olds' memory for action sequences could be reinstated by watching an experimenter perform half of the activities learned in initial training.

Although research on reenactment and physical reinstatement has focused on preschool children, there is a large body of research on verbal reinstatement with children at all ages as well as adults. In the adult literature, verbal rehearsal has been shown to enhance recall, presumably by reinforcing memory traces and strengthening memory representations (Linton, 1982; Rubin & Kozin, 1984). Several studies have shown that repeated verbal recall of past events can also improve children's recall. For example, when asked to recall creative movement workshops, preschool children remembered more information one month later if they had also been asked to recall the workshops in the same day as they occurred (Hudson, 1990a). However, in other studies where verbal rehearsal effects have been found, they have been isolated to cued recall (Goodman, Bottoms, Schwartz-Kenney, & Rudy, 1991), to free recall (Baker-Ward et al., 1990), or to older but not younger children (Gee & Pipe, 1995).

In a recent review, Fivush and Schwartzmueller (1995) argue that verbal rehearsal is effective only if adult questioning enables children to form a more coherent representation of a past event. If the event is already well represented, rehearsal may have little effect. If the event is not well represented, rehearsal may have an effect only if it is experienced many times and if the questioning assists children in forming a more complete or better organized event memory. Therefore, when children's verbal skills are limited, verbal exchanges may not serve as effective reminders (Hudson, 1990b, 1993a).

In general, research has shown that children of all ages are affected by experiences that both alter and strengthen event memories during storage. However, there is some evidence that younger children may be more susceptible to alterations in storage than older children. They have more difficulty distinguishing particular episodes of routine events, and, over time, they tend to recall more inaccurate information. Poole and White (1993) found that over a two-year delay, 6-, 8-, and 10-year-old children recalled more inaccurate event information (20%) than adults (7%) despite the fact that participants at all ages recalled equivalent levels of accurate information.

DEVELOPMENTAL DIFFERENCES IN MEMORY RETRIEVAL

As discussed above, research on children's use of deliberate retrieval strategies has yielded a large body of research documenting young children's inability to use deliberate retrieval strategies in directed memory tasks. However, memory for real-world events is assumed to be more automatic and less deliberate. Are there also developmental differences in children's ability to retrieve event memories, even in more naturalistic recall contents?

Evidence suggests that preschool children do, in fact, have greater difficulty in retrieving event memories as compared with older children. They often require more specific questioning or more specific cues to recall event information. For example, when specific questions are provided in addition to open-ended ones, younger children's recall improves significantly (Baker-Ward et al., 1993; Hudson, 1990a). In recalling a pediatric examination, three-year-olds recalled only 26% of the total number of features of the event, whereas five-year-olds recalled 42%, and seven-year-olds recalled 61%. When responses to specific questions were included, three-year-olds recalled 75% of the features as compared with 82% for both five- and seven-year-olds. Although age differences were still apparent, the differences were not as dramatic as those for responses to open-ended questions alone (Baker-Ward et al., 1993).

Studies in which children are given physical cues and props during memory retrieval have also found that age differences in recall dissipate with increased memory support (Fivush, Kuebli, & Clubb, 1992; Salmon, Bidrose, & Pipe, 1995; Smith, Ratner, & Hobart, 1987). Price and Goodman (1990) found that children from two to five years verbally recalled more about a novel event, visiting a "wizard," when they returned to the wizard's room and could view the associated props. Pipe and Wilson (1994) found that 6- and 10-year-old children who were shown props from an original experience recalled more information about a novel event with a magician both 10 days and 10 weeks later than did children who simply returned to the context (without props) or who did not receive any type of support. Interestingly, a recent study by Butler, Gross, and Hayne (1995) found that five- to six-year-old children who were asked to draw what happened during a trip to a fire station one day or one month in the past verbally recalled more information about the event than children who were simply asked to tell what happened. The activity of drawing may have provided children with additional retrieval cues or may have focused children's attention on the specific details of the experience rather than the more routine aspects.

These findings suggest that a large part of the age differences found in children's verbal recall are due to age differences in the ability to verbally report information. This conclusion is also supported by research comparing verbal and behavioral recall development. When behavioral reenactment is measured, two-and-a-half- and three-year-old children are able to recall as many actions from a novel event as five-year-olds, despite the fact that their verbal recall is much more limited (Fivush et al., 1992; Price & Goodman, 1990). Preschool children, in particular, will frequently act out, with props, actions that they are either unable or unwilling to recount verbally (DeLoache, 1995). This raises the issue of how much verbal recall is affected by children's language ability.

RELATIONS BETWEEN LONG-TERM MEMORY AND VERBAL EXPRESSION

Because children's ability to verbally recall events is important in real-world contexts such as classrooms and courtrooms, it is necessary to consider how children develop the skills to verbally report event memories. Several researchers (Hudson, 1990b; Nelson, 1990, 1993) have proposed that the development of narrative ability is critical to the ability to report event memories. Even though children at two and three years of age may have the language skills necessary to verbally encode events, they may have difficulty reporting event information because they do not possess narrative skills for verbally organizing a complete, coherent, and temporally sequenced account of an event.

Research on the development of narrative skills has examined how parents elicit memory narratives from children in conversations about shared past experiences. By participating in memory conversations, children learn the social value of reminiscing and also learn how to structure a memory narrative. Talking about past events may also serve to reinstate event memories (Hudson, 1990b; Nelson, 1993).

Two different elicitation styles have been identified in mother/child memory conversations (Fivush & Fromhoff, 1988; Hudson, 1993a; Reese & Fivush, 1993). Mothers who use an elaborative style add information to their children's responses, provide detailed memory cues, and volunteer their own memories of the event under discussion. Mothers who use a more repetitive style focus more on children's responses to specific memory questions and tend to ask numerous similar questions.

Maternal elicitation styles are associated with different levels of memory performance by preschool children. Children of elaborative parents provide more information and more specific details in mother/child memory conversations than do children of repetitive mothers (Fivush & Fromhoff, 1988; Hudson, 1990a, 1993b; Reese & Fivush, 1993). More importantly, differences in maternal elicitation style have long-term effects on children's narrative development. McCabe and Peterson (1991) found that two- to three-and-a-half-year-old children of elaborative mothers produced more coherent independent memory narratives one year later than did children of repetitive mothers. Reese, Haden, and Fivush (1993) found that the level of maternal elaboration at 40 months of age was positively correlated with the number of children's memory responses at 58 and 70 months. Presumably, these differences reflect different narrative skills that are taught by mothers using different elicitation styles. The elaborative style fosters more general narrative abilities, whereas the repetitive style teaches children how to answer specific memory questions but not how to organize full accounts on their own.

Of course, these data do not tell whether children of elaborative mothers actually remember more than children of repetitive mothers or whether they are simply better able to report what they remember. In addition, research has shown that young children recall more information about events both verbally and nonverbally when they are provided with external aids such as props or self-generated drawings (see above), suggesting that the conversational context may underestimate young children's recall (Bauer & Wewerka, 1997). However, given that verbal recall assessments are frequently used in both experimental and real-world contexts, it is difficult to distinguish event memory from verbal recall. Moreover, the ability to narrate an event memory without contextual support is an important milestone in the development of long-term memory regardless of whether it is the most sensitive measure of children's memory ability.

HOW LONG-TERM MEMORY DEVELOPS

It should be clear by now that there are dynamic relationships between encoding, storage, retrieval, and reporting processes. Nevertheless, the research reviewed here suggests that there are developmental differences in all of these aspects of memory that can contribute to children's ability to verbally recall events.

Brainerd and others (Brainerd & Reyna, 1990; Brainerd et al., 1990; Howe & Brainerd, 1989; Howe & O'Sullivan, 1997) analyzed the relative contributions of encoding, storage, and retrieval failures to processes of forgetting. Across a variety of memory tasks (e.g., memory for pictures, word lists, play events, object locations), storage failure contributed more to forgetting rates than did retrieval failure. Moreover, storage failure rates tended to decline with age from early childhood into adulthood, but the declines in retrieval failure were fairly modest. It remains to be seen whether this approach can be used to explain developmental differences in storage and retrieval across a greater array of memory tasks. In addition, the model does not yet specify the source of forgetting (e.g., decay, interference, blending) or whether there are developmental differences in different types of storage failure.

Approaching the question from a more macro level, theorists have argued that the sociocultural context in which memories about past events are discussed with young children as well as their emerging language skills allows children to construct more elaborated event memory representations across the preschool years (Fivush & Haden, 1997; Hudson, 1990b; Nelson, 1993). Before children are able to organize memories into narratives, their event memories are more fragmented and less easily retrieved. The ability to narrate events, however, alters the way children understand and encode events as well as the way they retrieve and report event memories.

Basic-level and macro-level explanations are not mutually exclusive. Developmental differences in world knowledge and language skills allow children to encode more information about events. Decreases in storage failures with age can affect the probability that event information will persist in storage intact. At the same time, developmental differences in narrative abilities may affect how all children verbally retrieve and report event memories.

Recall context, prior knowledge, and level of language development affect the manner in which long-term memories are encoded, stored, retrieved at a later time, and expressed. Further, there are recursive relationships between encoding, storage, retrieval, and reporting processes. For these reasons, long-term memory is probably best characterized as a dynamic system composed of complex and interdependent processes and functions. This perspective has important implications for clinicians who are interested in assessing and treating children with language disorders.

CLINICAL IMPLICATIONS

There is relatively little clinical advantage in attempts to separate memory processes and functions in assessment or to try to independently treat these processes and functions in intervention. Rather, assessment and intervention should reflect the multifaceted nature of language and cognition as they co-occur in interpersonal and academic contexts. The assessment and intervention practices discussed below should illuminate the dynamic relationships between encoding, storage, recall, and reporting processes and the ways these processes transact with demands and constraints in the child's environment.

When we assess the interactions between language and memory, we are interested in the variability of the child's performance within and across conversational and/or academic memory contexts. At minimum, three questions guide assessment practices:

1. How much variation exists in children's long-term memories across recall contexts?
2. How does the child's memory vary in relationship to the nature of the information to be recalled?
3. What approaches effectively facilitate recall?

The assessment process is begun by asking parents, caregivers, and/or teachers to tell about two or three recent significant or novel experiences the child has been involved in (e.g., trips to the physician, an amusement park, or a relative's house; attendance at a party or concert; participation in a class field trip or a science project). Parents are asked about the level of the child's involvement in the experience, the kinds of memory supports that were provided (explanations, questions, discussion, review of photographs at a later time, etc.), and the opportunities the child has had to talk about the events since the time they occurred. Parents, caregivers, and/or teachers are also asked to tell in what activities or subjects the child is most interested. This kind of information is very useful for planning assessment and intervention activities that are related to children's prior knowledge and experiences.

We want to obtain evidence about children's long-term event memory in familiar and unfamiliar contexts. For the familiar context, we ask parents, caregivers, or teachers to make an audiotape of a conversation with the child in which they try to elicit the child's recall of a recent event. We are interested in the kind of elicitation style the adults use. Do they use an elaborative style in which they add information, provide memory cues, or discuss their own reflections? Do they use a repetitive style in which they pose a series of rephrased questions? We are also interested in the children's reports. Is their initial description complete, coherent, and understandable to someone who did not experience the situation? Do they provide specific details about the experience upon questioning?

Later, when the parents, caregivers, or teachers are not present, we ask children to tell about the same event they had discussed with the familiar adult. Because examiners are almost always strangers, this serves as an unfamiliar context. We want to know if children report the event more or less completely when they are talking to a listener who was not present when it occurred. This context also enables observations of the way children respond to clarification questions from unfamiliar adults.

We have devised a four-activity memory protocol for use in both assessment and intervention (see Figure 1). This protocol can help in planning assessment situations designed to answer assessment questions that concern memory for different kinds of information and facilitative strategies. Similarly, the protocol can be used in intervention for designing contexts that facilitate interactions between long-term memory and language. In both assessment and intervention, we recommend using a transdisciplinary approach (Patterson & Gillam, 1995). Clinicians should collaborate with parents, caregivers, or teachers to plan novel activities and corresponding recall procedures that include various combinations of the facilitative factors that were discussed in the preceding sections of this chapter.

In assessing or treating preschoolers, we work with parents and caregivers to implement a variety of interesting and unusual experiences

Facilitation Strategies	Activities			
	1	2	3	4
Prior to the activity				
Provide background information				
During the activity				
Explain the procedure				
Ask questions				
Increase level of participation				
Immediately after the activity				
Summarize what happened				
Ask recall questions				
At time of recall				
Reenactment				
Reinstatement				
Physical cues/props/photographs				
Child drawings				
Adult elaborations on recall				

Figure 1. A memory facilitation assessment and intervention chart.

that can be presented to the child on different days. We also plan six clarification questions to accompany each activity. Parents or caregivers elicit children's memory of each experience as soon as it is completed as well as one and two days later.

One parent/child pair we worked with recently chose to plant flowers, bake cookies, read a book, and make a simple art project together. For the first activity (planting flowers), the adult did not use any facilitating strategies before, during, or after the experience. Three days later, the parent and child baked cookies together. The adult used facilitating strategies before and during the activity but did not use any facilitating strategies during recall. The parent asked questions as she read the story, then she summarized the story immediately after reading. She used reenactment with toys, reinstatement, and pictures from the book during the three recall tasks. For their last activity, the parent and child made a valentine for the child's father. The adult did not use any memory facilitation strategies before, during, or after the activity, but she used photographs, child drawings, and elaboration strategies to facilitate questioning and recall.

In this case, there was a good deal of variation in the amount of recall across the four tasks. The child's performance in Activity 1 (planting flowers) was very much like his performance in Activity 4 (valentine card). Using facilitating strategies only at the time of recall was no better than not using any strategies at all. However, the child remembered more information, used higher level language, and answered more questions correctly when the parent used facilitating strategies during the activity and at the time of recall. The parent in this case was very interested in planning additional activities to test differences between the facilitating strategies, and we were happy to assist her in this effort. After a month of consulting with us and working with her child, this parent discovered that her child responded best when she asked questions during activities and immediately after activities. This case demonstrates how dynamic assessment practices become dynamic intervention practices as well.

We follow a very similar procedure when we assess and treat school-age children. In keeping with our transactional approach to assessment and intervention, we design the activities in collaboration with classroom teachers and other special educators. For example, recall the explanations given by a girl named Jennifer at the beginning of this chapter. The memory activities that were selected for Jennifer involved describing how to saddle a horse, retelling a story, learning and explaining a new game, and explaining a science concept (requirements of floating objects). In Jennifer's case, the facilitative strategies of prompting and child drawings just before recall and questioning during recall were the techniques to which she was the most responsive.

•   •   •

In summary, practitioners who are interested in communicative abilities in social and academic settings should not ignore relationships between memory and language. In fact, we have made the case that long-term memory is best considered to be a dynamic, complex system in which internal cognitive and linguistic processes interact recursively with environmental constraints and demands. This account of long-term memory challenges clinicians to provide intervention in contexts where it is necessary for successful functioning.

The dynamic facilitative strategy described above results in a seamless transition between assessment and intervention. For preschool-age children, practitioners demonstrate strategies (Figure 1) to parents and caregivers for use at home and in the child-care environment. In school settings, practitioners can use the facilitation strategies in lessons with entire classrooms, or they may teach regular educators to use the strategies in their teaching. In either case, children whose academic problems lie at the intersection between language and memory will benefit from teaching practices that enhance interactions between encoding, storage, retrieval, and reporting functions.

REFERENCES

Baker-Ward, L., Gordon, B.N., Ornstein, P.A., Larus, D.M., & Clubb, P.A. (1993). Young children's long-term retention of a pediatric examination. *Child Development, 64,* 1519–1533.

Baker-Ward, L.E., Hess, T.M., & Flannagan, D.A. (1990). The effects of involvement on children's memory for events. *Cognitive Development, 5,* 55–70.

Bauer, P.J., & Wewerka, S.S. (1997). Saying is revealing: Verbal expression of event memory in the transition from infancy to early childhood. In P. van den Broek, P.J. Bauer, & T. Bourg (Eds.), *Developmental spans in event comprehension and representation: Bridging fictional and actual events* (pp. 139–168). Hillsdale, NJ: Lawrence Erlbaum Associates.

Brainerd, C.J., & Reyna, V.F. (1990). Gist is the grist: Fuzzy-trace theory and the new intuitionism. *Developmental Review, 10,* 3–47.

Brainerd, C.J., Reyna, V.F., Howe, M.L., & Kingma, J. (1990). The development of forgetting and reminiscence. *Monographs of the Society for Research in Child Development, 55.*

Butler, E., Gross, J., & Hayne, H. (1995). The effect of drawing on memory performance in young children. *Developmental Psychology, 31,* 597–608.

Campbell, B.A., & Jaynes, J. (1966). Reinstatement. *Psychological Review, 73,* 478–480.

DeLoache, J.W. (1995). The use of dolls in interviewing young children. In M.S. Zaragoza, J.R. Graham, G.C.N. Hall, R. Hirschman, & Y.S. Ben-Porath (Eds.), *Memory and testimony in the child witness* (pp. 160–178). Thousand Oaks, CA: Sage Publications.

Farrar, M.J., & Goodman, G.S. (1990). Developmental differences in the relation between scripts and episodic memory: Do they exist? In R. Fivush & J.A. Hudson (Eds.), *What young children remember and why* (pp. 30–64). New York: Cambridge University Press.

Fivush, R., & Fromhoff, F.A. (1988). Style and structure in mother-child conversations about the past. *Discourse Processes, 11,* 337–355.

Fivush, R., & Haden, C.A. (1997). Narrating and representing experience: Preschoolers' developing autobiographical recounts. In P. van den Broek, P.J. Bauer, & T. Bourg (Eds.), *Developmental spans in event comprehension and representation: Bridging fictional and actual events* (pp. 169–198). Hillsdale, NJ: Lawrence Erlbaum Associates.

Fivush, R., Haden, C., & Adam, S. (1995). Structure and coherence of preschoolers' personal narratives over time: Implications for childhood amnesia. *Journal of Experimental Child Psychology, 60,* 32–56.

Fivush, R., & Hamond, N.R. (1989). Time and again: Effects of repetition and retention interval on 2 year olds' event recall. *Journal of Experimental Child Psychology, 47,* 259–273.

Fivush, R., Kuebli, J., & Clubb, P. (1992). The structure of events and event representations: A developmental analysis. *Child Development, 63,* 188–201.

Fivush, R., & Schwartzmueller, A. (1995). Say it once again: Effects of repeated questions on children's event recall. *Journal of Traumatic Stress, 8,* 555–580.

Foley, M.A., & Johnson, M.K. (1985). Confusions between memories for performed and imagined actions. *Child Development, 56,* 1145–1155.

Gee, S., & Pipe, M.E. (1995). Helping children to remember: The influence of object cues on children's accounts of a real event. *Developmental Psychology, 31,* 746–758.

Goodman, G.S., Bottoms, B.L., Schwartz-Kenney, B.M., & Rudy, L. (1991). Children's testimony about a stressful event: Improving children's reports. *Journal of Narrative and Life History, 1,* 69–99.

Goodman, G.S., Quas, J.A., Batterman-Faunce, J.M., Riddlesberger, M.M., & Kuhn, J. (1994). Predictors of accurate and inaccurate memories of traumatic events experienced in childhood. *Consciousness and Cognition, 3,* 269–294.

Howe, M.L. (1995). Interference effects in young children's long-term retention. *Developmental Psychology, 31,* 579–596.

Howe, M.L., & Brainerd, C.J. (1989). Development of long-term retention. *Developmental Review, 9,* 302–340.

Howe, M.L., Courage, M.L., & Bryant-Brown, L. (1992). Reinstating preschoolers' memories. *Developmental Psychology, 29,* 854–869.

Howe, M.L., Courage, M.L., & Peterson, C. (1995). How can I remember when "I" wasn't there: Long-term retention of traumatic experiences and emergence of the cognitive self. *Consciousness and Cognition, 3,* 327–355.

Howe, M.L., & O'Sullivan, J.T. (in press). What children's memories tell us about recalling our childhoods: A review of storage and retrieval processes in the development of long-term retention. *Psychological Review.*

Howe, M.L., O'Sullivan, J.T., & Marche, T.A. (1992). Toward a theory of the development of long-term retention. In M.L. Howe, C.J. Brainerd, & V.F. Reyna (Eds.), *Development of long-term retention* (pp. 245–255). New York: Springer-Verlag.

Hudson, J.A. (1990a). Constructive processes in children's event memory. *Developmental Psychology, 26*, 180–187.

Hudson, J.A. (1990b). The emergence of autobiographical memory in mother-child conversation. In R. Fivush & J.A. Hudson (Eds.), *Knowing and remembering in young children* (pp. 166–196). New York: Cambridge University Press.

Hudson, J.A. (1991). Learning to reminisce: A case study. *Journal of Narrative and Life History, 1*, 293–324.

Hudson, J.A. (1993a). Reminiscing with mothers and others: Autobiographical memory in young two-year-olds. *Journal of Narrative and Life History, 3*, 1–32.

Hudson, J.A. (1993b). Understanding events: The development of script knowledge. In M. Bennett (Ed.), *The child as psychologist* (pp. 142–167). London: Simon & Schuster.

Hudson, J.A., & Fivush, R. (1991). As time goes by: Sixth graders remember a kindergarten experience. *Applied Cognitive Psychology, 5*, 347–360.

Hudson, J.A., & Nelson, K. (1986). Repeated encounters of a similar kind: Effects of familiarity on children's autobiographic memory. *Cognitive Development, 1*, 253–271.

Hudson, J.A., & Sheffield, E.G. (in press). Déjà vu all over again: The effects of reenactment on 18-month-olds' event memory. *Child Development.*

Kail, R.V. (1989). *The development of memory in children* (2nd ed.). New York: W.H. Freeman & Co.

Linton, M. (1982). Transformations of memory in everyday life. In U. Neisser (Ed.), *Memory observed* (pp. 77–92). San Francisco: W.H. Freeman & Co.

McCabe, A., & Peterson, C. (1991). Getting the story: A longitudinal study of parental styles in eliciting narratives and developing narrative skill. In A. McCabe & C. Peterson (Eds.), *Developing narrative structure* (pp. 217–253). Hillsdale, NJ: Lawrence Erlbaum Associates.

Myles-Worsley, M., Cromer, C.C., & Dodd, D.H. (1986). Children's preschool script reconstruction: Reliance on general knowledge as memory fades. *Developmental Psychology, 22*, 22–30.

Nelson, K. (1990). Remembering, forgetting, and childhood amnesia. In R. Fivush & J.A. Hudson (Eds.), *Knowing and remembering in young children* (pp. 301–316). New York: Cambridge University Press.

Nelson, K. (1993). The psychological and social origins of autobiographical memory. *Psychological Science, 4*, 7–14.

Nelson, K. (1994). Long-term retention of memory for preverbal experience: Evidence and implications. *Memory, 2*, 467–475.

Ornstein, P.A., Gordon, B.N., & Larus, D.M. (1992). Children's memory for a personally experienced event: Implications for testimony. *Applied Cognitive Psychology, 6*, 49–60.

Ornstein, P.A., Larus, D.M., & Clubb, P.A. (1991). Understanding children's testimony: Implications of research on the development of memory. *Annals of Child Development, 8*, 145–176.

Ornstein, P.A., Shapiro, L.R., Clubb, P.A., Follner, A., & Baker-Ward, L. (1996). The influence of prior knowledge on children's memory for salient medical experience. In N. Stein, P.A. Ornstein, B. Tversky, & C.J. Brainerd (Eds.), *Memory for everyday and emotional events* (pp. 83–111). Hillsdale, NJ: Lawrence Erlbaum Associates.

Patterson, S., & Gillam, R.B. (1995). Team collaboration in the evaluation of language in students above the primary grades. In D.F. Tibbits (Ed.), *Language intervention: Beyond the primary grades* (pp. 137–182). Austin, TX: PRO-ED.

Pillemer, D.B., Picariello, M.L., & Pruett, J.C. (1994). Very long-term memories of a salient childhood event. *Applied Cognitive Psychology, 8*, 95–106.

Pipe, M.E., & Wilson, C. (1994). Cues and secrets: Influences on children's event reports. *Developmental Psychology, 30*, 515–525.

Poole, D.A., & White, L.T. (1993). Tell me again and again: Stability and change in the repeated testimonies of children and adults. In M. Zaragoza (Ed.), *Memory, suggestibility, and eyewitness testimony in children and adults* (pp. 24–43). New York: Harper & Row.

Price, D.W.W., & Goodman, G.S. (1990). Visiting the wizard: Children's memory for a recurring event. *Child Development, 61*, 664–680.

Reese, E., & Fivush, R. (1993). Parental styles of talking about the past. *Developmental Psychology, 29*, 596–606.

Reese, E., Haden, C.A., & Fivush, R. (1993). Mother-child conversations about the past: Relationships of style and memory over time. *Cognitive Development, 8*, 403–430.

Rubin, D.C., & Kozin, M. (1984). Vivid memories. *Cognition, 16*, 81–95.

Rudy, L., & Goodman, G.S. (1991). Effects of participation on children's reports: Implications for children's testimony. *Developmental Psychology, 27*, 527–538.

Salmon, K., Bidrose, S., & Pipe, M.E. (1995). Providing props to facilitate children's event reports: A comparison of toys and real items. *Journal of Experimental Child Psychology, 601*, 174–195.

Schneider, W., & Bjorklund, D.F. (in press). Memory. In R.S. Sigler & D. Kuhn (Eds.), B. Damon (General Ed.), *Handbook of child psychology: Cognitive, language, and perceptual development* (Vol. 2). New York: John Wiley & Sons.

Shapiro, L.R., Clubb, P.A., & Ornstein, P.A. (1995). *The effect of knowledge on children's memory reports for their five-year-old checkups.* Paper presented at the meeting of the Society for Research in Child Development, Indianapolis, IN.

Sheffield, E.G., & Hudson, J.A. (1994). Reactivation of toddlers' event memories. *Memory, 2*, 447–465.

Smith, B.S., Ratner, H.H., & Hobart, C.J. (1987). The role of cueing and organization in children's memory for events. *Journal of Experimental Child Psychology, 44*, 1–24.

Tessler, M., & Nelson, K. (1994). Making memories: The influence of joint encoding on later recall by young children. *Consciousness and Cognition, 3*, 307–326.

8

Making It Hang Together: Children's Use of Mental Frameworks To Structure Narratives

Rita C. Naremore

Three-year-old Caitlin ran into the kitchen from the backyard, where she had been playing. "Mom, Mom," she said, "there's a big tiger in the backyard and Phillip is chasing it and we're building a fort." With this, she ran out again, slamming the door behind her. Caitlin was using language to construct a ministory, building on what Halliday (1975) called the *informative function*. Halliday maintained that the informative function, or the use of language to tell other people something they do not already know, appears soon after the child is able to construct propositional utterances. Caitlin's motivation and ability to inform other people about her own world will lead her to narratives. *Narrative* will be used here as a generic term including extended accounts of events, descriptions, stories, and all the other formats children use to turn their experiences and fantasies into textual language.

NARRATIVES AND MENTAL FRAMEWORKS

Many of the narratives told by children and adults are mapped onto knowledge about the world that comes from experience, either firsthand (based on direct participation in an event) or secondhand (based on reading about or hearing about an event). Schank and Abelson (1977) proposed that, from memories, people can construct scripts, which are integrated, organized, stereotypical mental representations of everyday events. Adults

Top Lang Disord 1997;18(1):16–31
© 1997 Aspen Publishers, Inc.

can construct scripts for making scrambled eggs, calling 911 to report an emergency, attending a wedding, and participating in hundreds of other events about which they have experienced or learned. Children, whose experience with the world is more limited, may have fewer or less elaborate scripts than adults (Fivush & Slackman, 1986; Nelson, 1978; Nelson & Gruendel, 1981), but they also construct scripts for events such as getting ready for bed, going to school, or going to a birthday party. The scripts constructed for various events allow people to anticipate what will probably happen when encountering a new instance of an event encountered in the past. For example, a child's school script will allow him or her to anticipate the presence of a teacher in the classroom when he or she begins a new grade. In addition, scripts serve as frameworks when people organize verbal accounts of scripted events or when they comprehend other people's accounts. For example, if a speaker is talking about scrambling eggs and cooking bacon, it is assumed he or she is talking about breakfast, and listeners interpret other parts of the narrative in this context.

The idea of a framework, or frame, will be important to the subsequent discussion of the relations between long-term memory (LTM) and narrative. In its most literal sense, a framework is a supporting structure for some larger construction. As the term is used here, a *framework* (or *frame*—the two terms will be used interchangeably) is a mental structure formed from experience, used both as a support for recall and retrieval of information and as a support for narratives incorporating this information. A script is one such narrative framework, but there are others.

In addition to constructing scripted event representations from memories, people also develop other frameworks for organizing narratives. One of these has been called *story grammar* (Stein & Glenn, 1979). While scripts are mental representations of world knowledge, story grammars are mental frameworks used for comprehending and organizing those particular forms of narratives called *stories*. In this sense, a story might be called a *rhetorical framework* (Kintsch, 1988).

Every culture has its own understanding of how to tell a story. In mainstream American culture, stories are expected to have certain characteristics. Americans expect stories to be "about something," or to be goal oriented. They expect stories to have a setting (the place and time of the story) and characters. Americans also expect stories to be organized in terms of episodes. An episode consists of an initiating event (something to which the story's characters must respond), an attempt by the characters to respond to the event, and a consequence of their attempt. Stories may have one or many episodes. When the episodes are completed, Americans expect an ending, letting them know that the story is over. People develop ideas about what a story should be like as a result of hearing (or reading) stories. By the time they begin school, many children have well-developed story frameworks that they can use to structure stories they tell themselves and to understand stories told by other people.

COMBINING SCRIPT AND STORY FRAMEWORKS

It is easier for children to comprehend and tell stories that are not only organized around a story framework but also based on their scripted event representations (Applebee, 1978; Pace & Feagans, 1984; Stein, 1979). The combination of a script and a story framework seems to provide a powerful organizing tool for a child, and many of the stories in children's early reading texts are organized around events for which a child might be assumed to have a script. The power of this combination for a child's own story construction can be seen in the following two stories told by a kindergartner named Chris. To elicit the first story, we asked Chris to tell a story about a boy who was afraid of the dark. We knew Chris had a script for such a story because his parents reported that he has a little brother who asks to have the light left on every night.

> Once there was a boy who was afraid of the dark. He saw monsters under his bed and in his closet and everywhere. So he called his mom, and she came and shined a flashlight and told him no monsters lived in his room. And he went to sleep. The end.

For the second story, Chris was asked to tell a story about a boy who took care of his father's sheep. It was assumed that Chris had no "shepherding" script, living as he does in the city.

> Once there was a boy who took care of his father's sheep. He gave them water to drink. He gave them grass to eat. He made sure wolves didn't eat them. He put them in the barn at night. The end.

The first story contains a clear episode: initiating event (he saw monsters), attempt (he called his mom), and consequence (she told him there were no monsters). The second story consists of a list of tasks performed by the boy, revealing little or no episodic structure. When Chris is unable to call on a script to support his narrative, he seems unable to use his story framework as well.

Why are script frames and story frameworks such powerful structures for children's narratives? How are they formed? How does the child access them for use in composing and comprehending narratives? How can speech-language pathologists (SLPs) determine whether a child can use narrative frameworks? These are questions to be addressed in the remainder of this chapter.

NARRATIVE FRAMEWORKS AND LONG-TERM MEMORY

The theoretical framework used in this section is derived from the work of Kintsch and his associates (Ericsson & Kintsch, 1991; Kintsch, 1988, 1992, 1994; van Dijk & Kintsch, 1983). Ericsson and Kintsch (1991) conceive of long-term memory as being like the universe, in which there are galaxies of knowledge about various topics, with subclusters like star systems. Information within a subcluster contains local structure (such as chronological order) as well as some very specific relations (such as cause-effect relationships). Information about a topic is retrieved from such a knowledge base via a generate-edit process involving the use of retrieval cues (Kintsch, 1987). A cue has several components: contextual features, constraints imposed by the text type and audience, and content specifications. For example, a request to tell a friend about a baseball game seen yesterday contains contextual features (you and your friend are in some place at some time), text type and audience features (you are going to give an account of a game you witnessed to a familiar audience), and content specifications (you are going to tell about a specific baseball game). Another retrieval cue might cause you to go into the same content domain but pull up different information. For example, the request to tell a foreign visitor how baseball is played would result in the retrieval of different baseball-related information. Given the retrieval cue, a search is made of existing knowledge. This search is made automatically, generally without a conscious effort. Based on the search of LTM, ideas are generated and are then organized.

Both content and form may provide a basis for organizing a text. The nature of the ideas themselves may determine the organization. According to Kintsch (1987), ideas are always interrelated in some way in LTM. Sometimes these interrelationships are strong, direct, and quite unique, as in a script specifying the events in a game such as baseball. If a script applies to a given set of ideas, it is usually quite clear what follows what in the text. On the other hand, when a particular body of content can be organized in many different ways, formal rhetorical strategies (such as those needed for stories, arguments, etc.) then become important to the organization process. Kintsch (1987) proposes that "when people have a choice, they tend to select the largest possible unit to organize a text. That is, if there is a suitable frame, that is used; but if no frame fits the text, people still organize the text, but in terms of smaller, propositional units" (p. 169). In other words, the largest, or most general, frame appropriate to the content is the most likely to be used in organizing the narrative.

To clarify this, think again about the two requests to talk about baseball presented above: (1) to tell about a specific baseball game and (2) to tell about how to play baseball. When competent adults tell how to play baseball, a conventional framework is used (i.e., listeners have certain expectations about how the description will be given). As Klann-Delius (1987) discovered, these include how to carry out the moves in the game, the starting point and goal of the moves, and the interrelationships among the moves. This set of expectations is a part of the "how to play a game" framework of most adults, and this frame will tend to govern explanations of how to play all games.

On the other hand, there are many possible ways to organize a narrative about a specific baseball game. One might, for example, begin with telling who won and then explain how the runs were scored, or one might choose to organize the narrative around the actions of one individual player. Kintsch (1987) suggests that, in this situation, the largest applicable frame to organize the narrative is generally used. If the instruction is to tell a story about a baseball game, then the story framework, being the largest (most general) frame, will organize the narrative. However, if there is an argument about the baseball game, then the typical strategies for argument (make a point, then give evidence to support the point) will organize the talk about the game. If the cue for the narrative is simply "tell me about the game," then people will tend to use their baseball script to organize the narrative. If one does not have a script framework to use, then one will look for other organizational schemes, at the level of what Kintsch calls *propositional units,* such as a focus on an individual player's actions.

THE CASE OF THE CHILD

Consider the case of a child who is asked to "make up a story about a soccer game." Before taking the child faced with this narrative task on a journey through his or her LTM, it might be useful to think about the LTM space the child will traverse. This space might be visualized as being organized like a tree diagram, with nodes hierarchically arranged, as seen in Figure 1.

The "soccer" node leads to several other nodes, each of which in turn leads to more and more specific information. Somewhere in this body of content, there exists a script for how to play soccer. In addition, probably at a level higher than any content node, there is a node for textbase information, in which the organizational patterns for stories, arguments, and so forth are stored. Elsewhere in LTM are the syntactic and phonological rules of English, together with the dictionary of word meanings known by this child. The child's journey through this space in response to the request to "make up a story about a soccer game" is almost certainly a matter of simultaneous processing. Even though speakers are forced to talk about the process as though it occurred in steps from first to last, it is likely that many nodes will be accessed at once. The process might be something like the following.

Since the child has been asked to "make up a story about a soccer game," the textbase node for stories would be activated along with the

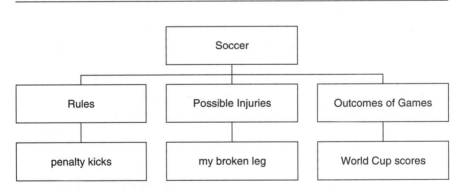

Figure 1. A partial LTM node for soccer information.

node for soccer scripts, giving the child two organizationally relevant constraints to work with in calling up the content nodes. The story frame could provide an overall organizational frame, causing the child to search for likely characters and problems related to soccer games. For example, the child might retrieve information about soccer injuries or about exciting games won at the last minute. The soccer script would be needed to help frame the chronological and hierarchical relations of smaller story units. If the child's story is to contain an account of an imaginary game, the soccer script would be needed to help the child organize this account. The story and script frames would constrain the search of the "soccer" content node, helping the child to decide which soccer-related information is relevant to the narrative. How does the child know which story and script nodes to activate? This depends entirely on the child's comprehension of the request (or, in Kintsch's terms, the nature of the retrieval cue). Presumably, the child's understanding of this cue is part of pragmatic and meta-linguistic knowledge.

The cues for accessing what is stored in LTM, then, are both contextual ("tell me a story . . .") and informational (what do you know about playing soccer?). Not all of the information about soccer in the child's LTM will be relevant (the scores of the last two World Cup soccer games may be unimportant to the story the child is constructing). How does the child know which pieces of his content knowledge will be relevant? This appears to depend to a certain extent on the scripts and schemata constructed for the purpose of the narrative in a particular context. The child uses the structure of his soccer script and the framework of his potential story (e.g., a story about a boy who saves his team's chance at the championship by making a heroic play) as cues for accessing particular long-term information structures. The knowledge about how scripts are organized and how stories are constructed then becomes separate pieces of information to be accessed. As the child narrows the focus of the search in terms of the specific story framework and script needed for the narrative at hand, the rest of the search will be organized, and this organization can then be used by the child to generate a narrative.

ASSESSING CHILDREN'S USE OF NARRATIVE FRAMEWORKS

When assessing children's abilities to use their scripts and narrative frameworks to structure their comprehension and production of stories and events, it is important that the SLP approach the task with a clear sense of what information is needed to evaluate children's narrative competence. The following questions should guide the SLP's approach:

1. Does this child have experience with the event, so that a script might have been formed?
2. Can the child use the script to act out (without the necessity for language) a narrative about the event?
3. Can the child compose a verbal account of the event?
4. Can the child retell a well-formed story involving the event?
5. Can the child answer factual recall and inferencing questions about the story?
6. Can the child compose a well-formed story built on the scripted event?

To show how these questions might govern an assessment task, we will recount an evaluation conducted with a kindergarten child, Toni. Toni was referred to the SLP, Ann, because she did not talk in the classroom and had difficulty following directions. The teacher asked that her hearing be checked and also suggested that a full evaluation be conducted to rule out any developmental disability. Toni's hearing was found to be unimpaired, and the narrative testing was a part of the larger evaluation designed to find the source of her classroom difficulties.

Experience with the event

As part of a questionnaire answered by Toni's mother, information about Toni's experience with several scripted events was gathered. A portion of the questionnaire follows (parents were to circle the appropriate response):

1. Does Toni go to the grocery store with you? Frequently Sometimes Never
2. Does Toni go to the library? Frequently Sometimes Never
3. Has Toni been to children's birthday parties? Frequently Sometimes Never
4. Does Toni have a bedtime routine (such as bath, tooth brushing, story, etc.)? Yes No
5. Please check any of the following food preparation tasks you would expect Toni to know how to do:

Making peanut butter and jelly sandwiches
Making a bowl of cereal with milk
Preparing a pizza in the microwave
Making scrambled eggs

This questionnaire was designed to find out what kinds of scripted event representations Toni might have, in addition to those she might have developed at school. Children of Toni's age almost certainly form scripts most readily for events they have experienced directly, as opposed to events they have read about or seen on television. Older children may have "secondhand" scripts, such as a script for traveling on a spaceship or a script for hunting a bear, based on books or television, but it is not wise to assume knowledge of such scripts for any child, especially for one who cannot yet read and has had limited exposure to school.

Demonstrating the event script

Toni's mother indicated that Toni frequently went with her to the grocery store, that she knew how to make peanut butter and jelly sandwiches and cereal with milk, and also that she had a regular bedtime routine. To check Toni's ability to represent her scripts for these events, Ann first put out the ingredients for a peanut butter and jelly sandwich, including a table knife, a loaf of bread, and jars of peanut butter and jelly. She asked Toni to make sandwiches for the two of them to share at snack time. Toni did this in an organized, if somewhat messy, fashion, demonstrating her ability to access a familiar script. Ann then took out a set of pictures she had made of a child getting ready for bed, including getting undressed, putting on pajamas, getting into bed, being kissed by the mother, having the light turned off, and seeing an imaginary monster looking in the window. She shuffled the pictures so that they were randomly arranged and asked Toni to put them in the right order.

Putting the script into words

Having established the presence and accessibility of Toni's scripts, Ann then set up a scenario for asking Toni to narrate her scripted event representations. The procedures generally used to probe for a child's narrative abilities are highly artificial. They are usually decontextualized, in that the child is asked to tell a story or to talk about some event in the absence of any communicative function and no realistically defined audience. Some children are sufficiently comfortable in these "performance" situations or are sufficiently willing to take risks, so they will readily participate. Other children become quite reticent, perhaps because they do not really understand what they are being asked to do or because they know something must be at stake here and they are not sure what the consequences of failure might be. To reduce the artificiality of the situation, it is important to provide the child with some understanding of who the audience for the narrative might be and with a reason for communicating to this audience. (See Kintsch, 1988; Naremore, Densmore, & Harman, 1995; and Pace & Feagans, 1984, for more extended discussions of these ideas.) The scenario used in this evaluation was as follows:

> Toni, I have a friend named Anna (shows picture of a young woman). She lives in Russia, but she is coming to America next week. She is going to babysit with my little boy while I go out to a movie. She doesn't have any children of her own, and she isn't quite sure what to do when it's bedtime for him. I thought I would make a tape for her, to help her know what little children do at bedtime, and I'd like you to help me. Here's my tape recorder. I'll start. Anna, first my little boy needs to get undressed and put on his pajamas. Now, you talk, Toni. What happens after he gets his pajamas on?

Ann does several appropriate things with this scenario. First, she specifies a realistic audience and a reason for talking to this person via a tape recorder. In addition, she begins the narrative herself, modeling the appropriate language conventions (the use of *you* with present tense verbs). Toni's scripted event recounting is shown below:

> You have to read a story. Then you have to go to the bathroom. Then you get into bed, and pull up the covers, and have a kiss goodnight. Then you go to sleep or maybe your mom rubs your back.

Toni's scripted event recounting is reasonably complete and coherent, indicating that she was able to access her script for this event and use it to structure the narrative. There are some script elements that might not be included in an adult's bedtime script, such as giving the child a back rub. Even though this might not be mentioned by an adult presenting this script, it is certainly not inappropriate to the event.

Retelling a story based on the script

Having obtained a scripted event account from Toni, Ann then turned her attention to Toni's use of story frameworks. She began by asking Toni some questions to investigate her background knowledge relevant to the story. Since the story was about a boy who was afraid of the dark at bedtime, she asked Toni whether she knew any "little kids" who were afraid of the dark when they went to bed. She then probed to find out whether the idea of seeing monsters or hearing ghosts was familiar to Toni. Toni reported that her sister used to be afraid of the dark and always wanted the light left on. She said her sister was afraid there was a robber in the closet who would come out and get her if the light was off. Having ascertained that the situation of being afraid of the dark at bedtime was a familiar one to Toni, Ann selected the book *Timothy and the Night Noises* (Dinardo, 1986) for her assessment of Toni's story framework knowledge. Although this step, appropriate text selection, is often omitted in assessment, it is a crucial one. As Kintsch (1994) pointed out, a child is not likely to comprehend a text unless the information provided in the text is based on some prior knowledge. While a child may be able to remember a text, in the sense of being able to repeat or summarize it, the child needs to truly understand a text, in the sense of being able to integrate it into existing knowledge structures or make inferences about it. The child's prior knowledge about the topic of the text (what the story is about) should be investigated prior to the time the story is chosen. Although it might be interesting to see what a child could do with a story about a totally unfamiliar topic, the first goal of assessment here is to provide a situation in which the child's optimal performance can be achieved. Thus, it is important to use a story the child can both understand and integrate with existing knowledge.

In addition to using prior knowledge about the topic to understand a story, children also use their knowledge of what a story is supposed to be like when they comprehend and narrate stories. As noted previously, story frameworks are stored in LTM for young children; the retrieval of a framework is presumably cued by the word *story* or by the presence of a book. Certain routines and phrases, such as *once upon a time*, are probably stored along with the frameworks. One aspect of a story assessment involves determining whether a child can retrieve a story framework and use it to retell an episodic story.

If a child has seldom heard stories or been read to, it is unlikely that a story framework exists in this child's LTM. Some probing to find out about the child's previous exposure to stories is appropriate if doubt exists about the child's literacy environment. If the child is unable to retell a well-formed story using its episodic structure, it is important to know whether this failure is due to the likely absence of a framework or to the inability to use a framework to structure a narrative. In this case, Ann knew that Toni had been to a year of preschool before kindergarten and that she had been read to in preschool, if not at home.

For the story retelling task, Ann sat beside Toni so that she might look at the pictures while the book was read. Ann then gave a copy of the book, with the print covered, to Toni, adding, "Now I'd like you to tell this story for my tape recorder, so some other child could listen to it. You can look at the pictures to help you remember what the story is about. I'll start: This story is called *Timothy and the Night Noises* and it is being told by Toni. Toni, how does this story begin?" Toni's retelling of the story is shown below:

> Mama told him that it was time to go to bed. She kissed him goodnight. She, um, he, mama said, I mean his brother said "mama don't turn off the lights." He said "all you are is a big baby." He heard a noise, OOOOOO. She said it was just the wind and she said "I'm going to stay in here for a little while." He rocked in the rocking chair to see if it was the rocking chair, and said, "there is a monster in here, little brother." It's just the noise of the tree. He finally tucked back into bed. Suddenly he feels something tapping on him. It was just his brother.

The original text of this story is presented in the Appendix, with the individual episodes identified. A comparison of Toni's retelling with the original will show that she left out a great deal of the story, despite having the pictures to serve as cues. In addition, her retelling is not a story, in that there is no introduction to the characters and no sense of how the story hangs together. This latter problem is due in large part to the fact that Toni's retelling is not episodically structured. She failed to tie together even one of the four initiating event (IE)–attempt (A)–consequence (C) sequences in the original story. For example, as can be seen in the Appendix, the first episode is structured as follows:

IE He heard a noise: WOOOOOO.
A   He called, "Mama, help me. It's a ghost."
C   Mama said, "It's not a ghost. It's only the wind." She tucked him
    in and sat with him for awhile.

Toni repeated the IE, saying, "He heard a noise, OOOOOO." She also repeated the C, saying, "She said it was just the wind and she said 'I'm going to
stay in here for a little while.'" However, she left out the A. In the next episode,
Timothy hears a noise (IE), asks "What's that?" and jumps into his mother's
lap (A). He is told that it is only the noise of the rocking chair and rocks it
himself to make sure (C). In her retelling, Toni repeated only the C (He
rocked in the rocking chair to see if it was the rocking chair). In other
words, Toni apparently did not use the organizational framework already
provided in the story to help her organize her retelling. It is as though she
attempted to tie her memory of the text to the pictures, and, in the process
she failed to comprehend the relations among the events in the text itself.

A comparison of Toni's retelling with that of Amber, another kindergarten girl, will show what Toni might have done with this story:

It's time to go to bed. His mom went up to the bedroom. Timothy had
trouble putting on his clothes. His mom said, "There." She tucked him
into bed, kissed him on the forehead. She turned off the light and shut the
door. He heard a spooky sound like booo, booo, booo. He hollered for his
mom. She came. She took him out of bed. She said, "There's no spooky
man." She tucked him in bed. "I'll just sit with you for right now and read
a book." He heard another spooky sound. She said, "It's just the rocking
chair." He jumped into her lap just to check it out. Then he got back in
bed, and she tucked him back in. [Etc.]

Although space does not permit Amber's complete retelling of the story, it
is clear that Amber used a story framework. Although Amber failed to
introduce the characters, she structured her story episodically and even
substituted her own language (such as *hollered, spooky*) for that used in the
book. For example, in the first episode, Amber gave the IE (He heard a
spooky sound like booo, booo, booo), the A (He hollered for his mom), and
the C (She came. She took him out of bed. She said, "There's no spooky
man"). She was equally adept at retelling the constituents of the rest of the
episodes.

When a child can reword a story as Amber has done while retaining the episodic structure, it is a clear sign that the story has been integrated into the child's prior knowledge base, indicating true comprehension of the text. It is not likely that Amber's recall of this lengthy story could be a result of simple word-by-word or sentence-by-sentence memorization. Not only had she heard it only once, but she modified some of its lexicon while retaining the author's intended meaning, and this meaning for her involved the episodic relationships of the original text. This is the essence of the advantage a story framework gives to a child.

Answering questions about the story

The story framework should also enable children to comprehend the relations among the events in a story, even if they are unable to reconstruct the framework in their retelling. In the case of Toni, who was unable to retell the story using the story framework, it would be important to assess her comprehension. Asking questions about the relations among events (such as, "What did Timothy do when he heard the scary sound?" or "Why did Timothy call his mama?") will help assess the child's ability to use the story framework in a task that is somewhat simpler than constructing a retelling. In Toni's case, her generally correct responses to a set of comprehension questions indicated that she could use the story framework for comprehension, even though she could not use it to structure her own retelling.

EXPLAINING THE ASSESSMENT RESULTS

Ascertaining that the child does not use a story framework to structure a story retelling or a script framework to structure an account of an event such as a trip to the zoo is not the end of the task. Some explanation for the child's failure will be needed to help focus appropriate intervention. The explanation will generally involve one of the following questions.

Are relevant frameworks present?

First, does the child have enough background knowledge about the narrative topic to have formed a script or a story framework? There are children who have little of the knowledge that is assumed by authors of children's storybooks. A child who has never been to a zoo or an amusement park, who does not routinely sit down with parents and siblings for a family meal, who has no bedtime or morning routine involving teeth brushing or face washing, for example, may be at a real disadvantage in encounters with the stories and narrative tasks often found in many primary-grade classrooms. SLPs have a responsibility to make certain that teachers and other school professionals understand the linguistic and metacognitive aspects of story comprehension and narrative construction. SLPs also might suggest ways to help children to employ scripts as well as ways to develop (even secondhand) other useful scripts. Exposing the child to many varied stories based on school-relevant scripts will aid in both script development and the story frameworks.

If the child is known to have scripts and story frameworks but is not employing these in comprehension and production tasks, a more difficult set of questions arises. Is the child's problem one of accessing the appropriate framework or one of attaching language to it?

Can the child access the frameworks and attach language to them?

It is not entirely clear why a child might have trouble accessing the appropriate framework (such as script or story), assuming that framework is stored in LTM. One possible difficulty might lie in the child's interpretation of the retrieval cue. This would probably be characterized as a language problem; that is, a child who did not understand that "Tell me how you make a sandwich" was a cue to retrieve a script would need to be taught something about what that request really meant. In the case of a child like Toni, who seemed able to use a story framework to aid her comprehension of the events in the story but was unable to use it to structure a story retelling, it would be useful to probe further to discover whether Toni understood the retelling task itself. Modeling the retelling, working with shorter stories, might be one way to proceed.

Another possible explanation to examine when a child's framework cannot be used to structure a spoken narrative is whether the child can attach language to the framework. In this case, the SLP needs to know first whether the child's difficulty is primarily a problem with word finding or perhaps a problem of inadequate vocabulary. Production and comprehension of cohesive, organized scripted event accounts and stories require a very specific set of words, such as conjunctions and relational adverbs, that are used to signal various sorts of relations among ideas in the narrative. Children with language impairment often have a limited number of such words and fail to comprehend the meanings of those they do use (Donahue & Bryan, 1984; Wiig & Semel, 1976). Helping children to understand the functions of these words in narratives and to increase their repertoires of relational terms often results in narratives that sound more coherent, reflecting the child's frameworks, and also results in more accurate mappings of relations in narratives the child hears or reads. When lack of needed vocabulary is not the source of the child's problem, it is necessary to search for other possible explanations, such as a more generalized difficulty with language processing.

Is limited processing capacity involved?

What can be said about a child who begins a narrative with what sounds like a script but then loses track of it and adds irrelevant details or stops altogether, as many children with language impairment do? Does this child lose the script framework somewhere in the process of constructing the narrative? In fact, this is entirely possible. If SLPs conceive of the language-impaired child's difficulty as being primarily one involving limited processing capacity, then it makes sense to say that the frame falls apart when the processing demands are greater than the child's capacity to handle them. Processing demands could include the following:

1. comprehending the retrieval cues (the instruction for what to do)
2. accessing the content
3. accessing the necessary framework (script or story)
4. using the frame to organize a search of the content
5. accessing the necessary vocabulary and syntax to encode the content, including linguistic expression of the requisite relations among parts of the content, while retaining the organizational frame

This processing breakdown explanation for a child's failure to use a script or story framework to organize a narrative is related to Westby's (1984) description of a child with a lack of planning and monitoring skills. Children with language impairment may have a limited command of syntax and morphology that is insufficient for automaticity. Thus, the cognitive demands of language tasks that other children handle with ease may overwhelm those who lack such metacognitive abilities.

To understand this problem, imagine that you have taken four years of college French in America but have never been to France. You have a reasonable vocabulary, you can construct sentences, and you understand what your teacher says. Then you go to France. First of all, everybody talks too fast. You can pick out words, but by the time you have figured out one sentence, the speaker is two sentences further. Then, when you try to talk, people look impatient, finish your sentences for you, or ask you to speak English. You are aware of how difficult it is to talk about places or events not present in the immediate context. All of your linguistic fluency appears to have deserted you as you struggle to remember the ending for a subjunctive verb. This is a bit like the situation the language-impaired children face in English. They, too, have vocabulary and syntax, but their ability to employ these in the service of communication is impaired, since they must expend cognitive energy figuring out how to say what they want to say.

This analogy should not be taken to mean that children are consciously trying to figure out how to say what they want to say. Indeed, they may not even be aware that their meaning is unclear. This is where the monitoring ability mentioned earlier enters. Proficient language users, when they talk or write or listen, are, on some level, serving as their own audiences. They hear themselves mispronounce a word and go back to correct it. They simplify an expression that might be too complex or decide to make an explanation more concise—and all of this is done on-line, while the communication is happening. As listeners or readers, they come to words they do not know and realize that they need to figure out what they mean or skip over them. They think about what the major points of the narrative are. All this is done while listening or reading is ongoing. Children with language impairment, who are struggling to fit vocabulary into sentence frames or to interpret the language used in a narrative, have little processing space for such ongoing monitoring activities. The simple act of constructing or comprehending meaningful utterances takes up too much room. Two goals are important for such children: (1) to help them achieve automaticity in the construction and comprehension of sentences and (2) to teach them to monitor their production and comprehension, even if it means slowing down their production and asking others to slow down as well.

•   •   •

Chris, age six, was talking with his four-year-old sister, Melanie:

What did you do at the zoo, Melanie?

We rode on the train and we saw the monkeys and one of them threw a banana peeling and hit another one on the head and they started to chase each other. And then we went to see the baby tiger, and then we got hot dogs and we ate outside.

Did you see any sharks?

Don't be silly. They don't have sharks at the zoo. Sharks are at the aquarium, and you have to go down the stairs so you can see underwater.

No, that's what you do to see the polar bears at the zoo.

You do it for the sharks too. We did it before when the baby shark was there. I remember everything better than you.

This may sound like a simple exercise testing a young child's memory about a trip to the zoo. In fact, Melanie is doing much more than remembering. She is calling up two scripted event frameworks, one for trips to the zoo and one for trips to the aquarium. She is using her frameworks to help structure a narrative—a scripted event account—for her brother. In the process, she is demonstrating her ability to access the frameworks, to encode them into language, and to use the knowledge cued by the frameworks to counter her brother's assertions in an argument. Melanie's mental frameworks are a powerful tool for her, and they will remain powerful as they are elaborated and as more frameworks, such as those needed for more elaborate stories and other narrative events, are formed.

One of the tasks of the SLP assessing the language ability of a school-age child is to determine how the child uses mental frameworks to structure narratives like Melanie's. Children who lack the ability to use mental frameworks are at a distinct disadvantage in comprehending and composing narratives, both spoken and written, in the classroom environment. When children fail to use presumably available frameworks to structure comprehension and production of narratives, it becomes important not only to discover the nature of the tasks on which children break down (e.g., giving a scripted event account or retelling a story), but also to identify the nature of the problem (e.g., lack of experience from which to construct a script or failure to monitor), so that appropriate intervention targets can be developed.

REFERENCES

Applebee, A. (1978). *The child's concept of story*. Chicago: University of Chicago Press.

Dinardo, J. (1986). *Timothy and the night noises*. New York: Simon & Schuster.

Donahue, M., & Bryan, T. (1984). Communicative skills and peer relations of learning disabled adolescents. *Topics in Language Disorders, 4*, 10–21.

Ericsson, K.A., & Kintsch, W. (1991). *Memory in comprehension and problem solving: A long-term working memory* (Institute of Cognitive Science Tech. Report. No. 91-13). Boulder, CO: University of Colorado.

Fivush, R., & Slackman, E. (1986). The acquisition and development of scripts. In K. Nelson (Ed.), *Event knowledge: Structure and function in development.* Hillsdale, NJ: Lawrence Erlbaum Associates.

Halliday, M.A.K. (1975). Development of texture in child language. In T. Myers (Ed.), *The development of conversation and discourse.* Edinburgh, Scotland: Edinburgh University Press.

Kintsch, W. (1987). Psychological processes in discourse production. In H. Dechert & M. Raupach (Eds.), *Psycholinguistic models of production.* Norwood, NJ: Ablex.

Kintsch, W. (1988). The use of knowledge in discourse processing: A construction-integration model. *Psychological Review, 95,* 163–182.

Kintsch, W. (1992). How readers construct situation models for stories: The role of syntactic cues and causal inferences. In A.F. Healy, S.M. Kosslyn, & R.M. Shiffrin (Eds.), *From learning processes to cognitive processes: Essays in honor of William K. Estes.* Hillsdale, NJ: Lawrence Erlbaum Associates.

Kintsch, W. (1994). Text comprehension, memory, and learning. *American Psychologist, 49,* 294–303.

Klann-Delius, G. (1987). Describing and explaining discourse structures: The case of explaining games. *Linguistics, 25,* 145–199.

Naremore, R.C., Densmore, A., & Harman, D. (1995). *Language intervention with school-aged children.* San Diego, CA: Singular Publishing.

Nelson, K. (1978). How young children represent knowledge in their world in and out of language. In R.S. Seigler (Ed.), *Children's thinking: What develops?* Hillsdale, NJ: Lawrence Erlbaum Associates.

Nelson, K., & Gruendel, J. (1981). Generalized event representations: Basic building blocks of cognitive development. In A. Brown & M. Lamb (Eds.), *Advances in developmental psychology* (Vol. 1). Hillsdale, NJ: Lawrence Erlbaum Associates.

Pace, A.J., & Feagans, L. (1984). Knowledge and language: Children's ability to use and communicate what they know about everyday experiences. In L. Feagans, C. Garvey, & R. Golinkoff (Eds.), *The origins and growth of communication.* Norwood, NJ: Ablex.

Schank, R.C., & Abelson, R.P. (1977). *Scripts, plans, goals, and understanding.* Hillsdale, NJ: Lawrence Erlbaum Associates.

Stein, N. (1979). How children understand stories: A developmental analysis. In L. Katz (Ed.), *Current topics in early childhood education* (Vol. 2). Norwood, NJ: Ablex.

Stein, N., & Glenn, C. (1979). An analysis of story comprehension in elementary school children. In R.O. Freedle (Ed.), *New directions in discourse processing.* Norwood, NJ: Ablex.

van Dijk, T.A., & Kintsch, W. (1983). *Strategies of discourse comprehension.* New York: Academic Press.

Westby, C.E. (1984). Development of narrative language abilities. In G.P. Wallach & K.G. Butler (Eds.), *Language learning disabilities in school-age children.* Baltimore: Williams & Wilkins.

Wiig, E., & Semel, E. (1976). *Language disabilities in children and adolescents.* Columbus, OH: Merrill.

Summary of the Text of *Timothy and the Night Noises,* by Jeffrey Dinardo, Simon & Schuster, 1986

Setting: Timothy and Martin (who are pictured as frogs, but who might just as easily be pictured as little boys) are getting ready for bed. Timothy has trouble getting his pajamas on, but his mother comes and helps. After his mother tucks them into bed, Timothy says he is afraid of the dark, but his mother tells him there is nothing to be afraid of, that his brother will be with him. After she turns off the light and leaves the room, Martin tells Timothy not to be a fathead. **Episode 1. (IE)** Then Timothy hears a "WOOO," and **(A)** yells for his mother, saying that he heard a ghost. **(C)** She assures him that it is only the wind. She sits with him for awhile. **Episode 2. (IE)** Then he hears another noise, "CREAK, CREAK." **(A)** He jumps into his mother's lap, saying, "What's that?" **(C)** She assures him that it is just the rocking chair, and he rocks it himself, just to be sure. **Episode 3. (IE)** As soon as he climbs back into bed, he sees something moving on the wall. **(A)** He calls for his mother, saying he sees a monster. **(C)** She says it is only the shadow of a tree on the wall and tucks him back into bed. **Episode 4. (IE)** After she leaves, Martin tells Timothy, "You're such a baby." Then the illustrations show a figure covered with a bedspread tapping Martin on the shoulder, saying "BOOO." (The reader must infer that it is Timothy.) **(A)** Martin runs out of the room, calling for his mother. **(C)** She comes back in with him, assuring him that there is no ghost. She tucks Martin in and turns to look at Timothy, who is fast asleep.

9

Accessing Long-Term Memory: Metacognitive Strategies and Strategic Action in Adolescents

M. Lorraine Wynn-Dancy and Ronald B. Gillam

During middle school and high school, adolescents invest much of their energies in sports. Successful athletes learn to play their sports strategically. Runners reserve their strength so they can forge ahead of the pack during the last quarter mile of a race. A baseball player may demonstrate strategic action by deliberately letting four pitches go by so that he or she can take a "base on balls" in order to load the bases for a powerful hitter who is next in the batting order. A power hitter may "swing for the fences" before he or she has any strikes but may just "try to make contact" if he or she already has two strikes.

Adolescents must also learn to employ strategies and strategic action to achieve success in school subjects. Throughout the elementary school years, teachers support students as they learn the fundamentals of reading, writing, and mathematical computation, and as they take the first steps toward learning *through* reading, writing, and mathematics. During the middle and high school years, there is an increase in the expectation for greater independence in academic learning. To be academically successful, adolescents must know how to acquire, store, recall, and use knowledge gained through assignments that are completed outside of class.

Preparation of this chapter was supported, in part, by a grant from the National Institute on Deafness and Other Communication Disorders to the second author.

Top Lang Disord 1997;18(1):32–44

Long-term memory plays an important role in this process. Students must store multiple pieces of information for retrieval during examinations, class discussions, and personal conversations. They must also master strategies for dealing with tasks that involve multiple and sequential problem-solving steps. Academic learning strategies can help students with lower capacities for memory and language increase their reading comprehension, remember what they have read for longer periods of time, and use their knowledge to complete classroom assignments successfully (Hasselhorn, 1995; Palinscar & Brown, 1984; Sawyer, Graham, & Harris, 1992). Unfortunately, as Pressley and Harris (1990) point out, many adolescents fail to automatically embrace suitable strategies for school success.

Strategies are effortful actions that are used to accomplish specific goals. Adolescents with language-based learning disabilities (LLD) often demonstrate inefficiency in applying effortful strategies toward learning academic material. Their deficiencies in utilizing controlled processes for memory recall and their poorer performance on memory tasks compared with their normally achieving peers have been well-documented (Ceci, Lea, & Ringstrom, 1980; Cooney & Swanson, 1987; Kail & Leonard, 1986; Swanson, 1986).

Nevertheless, it has been shown that students with LLD can improve their memory performance after receiving instruction in using organizational strategies (Dallago & Moeley, 1980; Graham, MacArthur, Schwartz, & Voth, 1992). In fact, McDaniel, Einstein, and Waddill (1990) point out that these adolescents often possess "sufficient resources to apply some effortful controlled strategies, but fail to use these strategies spontaneously" (p. 258).

This chapter describes two metacognitive strategies that influence long-term memory. One metacognitive strategy, called ARROW, promotes increased efficiency and accuracy in understanding and recalling information from expository texts. A second strategy, called BRIDGE, helps students organize information to support memory retrieval during classroom discussions.

Adolescents with LLD need to be taught to use learning strategies. However, it may be even more important for these students to learn to act strategically. It is not very likely that the formal strategies that are taught to students will apply to all of the learning situations they encounter. To be successful, adolescents need to set learning goals that are specific to each situation they face and to select steps in the strategies they know that will enable them to respond efficiently and effectively (Brown, 1989). To this end, a method is described for training the adolescent with LLD to formulate learning goals for each learning context, to look for similarities across past and present learning contexts, to consider the underlying features of strategies that have been successful in the past, and to apply those features to new learning contexts that may have different surface features but similar underlying structures and goals.

EFFORTFUL VERSUS AUTOMATIC METACOGNITION

Metacognition refers to processes through which individuals reflect on the demands inherent in a situation, the skills they bring to the task, and the actions that will need to be taken to ensure success. *Metacognitive processes* are ways of "thinking about thinking" in order to guide attention, memory, and planning resources.

Metacognition can be effortful or automatic. When metacognition is effortful, there is a voluntary, attentional focus on the cognitive demands associated with the context, the individual's goals with respect to the context, and the mental processes necessary to meet both the demands and the goals. In effortful metacognition, mental actions involve "the cognitive system's explicit knowledge of its own working" (Siegler & Shipley, 1995, p. 40).

When metacognition is automatic, mental processes are derived by a less conscious process (Flavell, 1985; Siegler & Shrager, 1984). As applied to learning, automatic metacognition involves selecting and using a problem-solving strategy at the moment a problem is encountered. The process of strategy selection can be so automatic that the student may be hard-pressed to explain how he or she went about solving a problem. This is similar to a kindergarten student who was able to solve auditory mathematical word problems that involved separate addition and multiplication steps. When the examiner asked this student how he arrived at his answers, he responded, "I don't know how to explain what I did. I just know I'm right." Clearly, this child had gone through some sort of mental problem-solving process in calculating answers to the questions. His problem-solving strategy was so automatic that he was not able to explain the process he used.

Many times, effortful and automatic strategies are used simply because they have been used before. For example, we have seen many LLD students approach a new assignment in exactly the same manner that they approached a previous assignment, even though the previous approach may have been unsuccessful. This is not an example of a strategic approach to problem solving.

Many successful students act strategically, however. They evaluate strategy outcomes with reference to the situations of use, and they make inferences about the likelihood of a strategy's effectiveness in new or different situations. According to Siegler and Shipley (1995), when learners think of a new strategy, the excitement of innovation sometimes catapults the strategy into a trial run, even though it may not have a proven track record. As more information is garnered about the new strategy's speed and accuracy, novelty decreases. The probability of a strategy's continued use is determined by its perceived effectiveness, its ease of use, and its relevance to the kinds of situations that are routinely encountered. Thus, speed, accuracy (effectiveness), relevance, and novelty are factors that influence strategy selection in problem solving. With practice, greater efficiency, and accuracy, strategies that were once effortful can become skills that are nearly automatic in some contexts.

When metacognitive strategy instruction is successful, some of the effortful strategies that are taught should gradually become automatic. However, intervention should not stop there. Naturalistic and experimental research suggests that when children first generate or learn a strategy, they may not evidence improvements in performance, a phenomenon known as a *utilization deficiency* (Bjorklund & Coyle, 1995). A similar situation occurs when performance is not increased after students begin to use an effortful strategy that they have been taught. Because utilization deficiencies have been observed naturally and experimentally, it is important that language specialists design instruction that includes strategy teaching, strategy implementation, and strategy generalization. Said another way, speech-language pathologists (SLPs) and other educators should select and teach metacognitive strategies they believe will be useful to the adolescents with whom they work. Once students know and can use the basic sequence of strategy steps, they should be taught how to select and use various steps in the effortful metacognitive strategies they know in order to meet the demands and learning goals associated with somewhat different learning situations.

EFFORTFUL STRATEGIES FOR IMPROVING LONG-TERM MEMORY

Many LLD adolescents have difficulty understanding and remembering expository texts. This is a very important problem because middle school and high school teachers expect students to acquire and retain information from outside reading assignments. The authors routinely teach two meta-cognitive strategies to adolescents. The first strategy, ARROW, was designed to help students with the long-term recall of information contained in reading assignments. The second strategy, BRIDGE, is a retrieval and organizational process for helping students access information from long-term memory for use in class discussions.

ARROW

ARROW stands for activate, read, reread, organize, and write. For the purposes of this chapter, assume that the ARROW strategy is being used with a group of adolescents who are studying the Santa Fe expedition. ARROW begins by teaching students how to *activate* and organize their prior knowledge (schema) about a subject. Activating prior knowledge has been shown to positively affect comprehension, learning, and long-term memory of information (Anderson & Pichert, 1978; Schmalhofer, 1995). Knowledge activation may be especially important for adolescents because there is some evidence that memory deficits in older children result from problems in accessing knowledge (Swanson, Reffel, & Trahan, 1991). According to Anderson (1994), prior knowledge acts as a sort of mental Velcro to which related, incoming information tends to stick. Prior knowledge also facilitates recall because it helps the learner determine what is or is not important. It provides an initial organizational structure that supports mental editing and reconstruction as new information arrives.

Initially, the students indicated that they had no relevant prior knowledge about the Santa Fe expedition. However, after a few minutes of discussion, most students realized that they already knew something about trading; about travel by horseback in the old West; and about the basic geography and climate of Texas, New Mexico, and Mexico. This is the kind of knowledge that needed to be activated so that new information could be readily added to it.

Wallach and Miller (1988) describe a number of knowledge activation and organization strategies. One favorite involves the following steps:

1. Read the title of the assignment. Ask yourself, "What are the key concepts in the title? What do I know about these concepts already?"
2. Write down the headings with four or five spaces between each entry. Ask yourself, "What does the author want me to learn?"

In this case, the title of the assignment in the students' text was "The Republic's Troubles with Mexico." Students identified the terms *Republic*, *Trouble*, and *Mexico* as key concepts. They knew already that *Republic* referred to the Republic of Texas, which was a government that no longer exists. They thought that *Trouble* probably referred to a war. Finally, they knew that *Mexico* was a nation that bordered the Republic of Texas and that Mexico was once much larger in size than it is today. Table 1 lists the headings from the text and the students' ideas about what they thought the author wanted them to learn.

Next, it is suggested that students *read* the assignment slowly. Students construct a mental representation of texts as they read (Foos, 1992). Encouraging and supporting the use of a slower reading rate gives students the time they need to construct a comprehensive representation of the text.

After students read the passage once slowly, it is suggested that they *reread* it at a faster rate. Rereading has been shown to enhance mental organization and recall (Jacoby, Levy, & Steinbach, 1992). In fact, Levy, Di Persio, and Hollingshead (1992) found that undergraduate college students continued to analyze the meaning of texts even on their fourth and fifth reread. The effects of rereading may be even greater if language specialists or students themselves revise the texts so that the language is more consistent with the individual student's language (McKeown, Beck, Sinatra, & Loxterman, 1992).

Carrell (1992) found that students who recalled more about expository texts organized their written recalls in a manner that was similar to the original texts. Therefore, students are asked to *organize* a text representa-

---

Table 1. Text headings from a social studies lesson on the Santa Fe expedition and student ideas about what the author wanted them to learn

Heading	Students' expectations
The Expedition Begins	When, why, and how the expedition started
Lost in the Canyon	How the people on the expedition got lost and how they found their way to Santa Fe
The Texans Surrender	What happened when the Texans fought the Mexicans and why they gave up
Imprisoned in Mexico City	How the Mexicans took the Texans to jail and how the Texans got out

tion by referring back to the list of headings they constructed during the activation step. In creating their first "textbase" (van Dijk & Kintsch, 1983), students should write at least two ideas under each heading. It is preferred that students generate this list from memory, but let them refer back to the text if necessary. The ideas that one student generated for each of the headings are listed in the box.

Finally, students are asked to use this organized outline to *write* a short summary of the passage. This positively affects long-term memory because it increases elaboration, serves as a rehearsal mechanism, and provides the opportunity for another rereading. This is one student's dictated summary:

> Mirabeau Lamar sent an expedition in 1841 to capture Santa Fe from Mexico and open trade there. The expedition got lost. Because of heat and lack of food and water, the Texans got sick and some of them died. As they got close to Santa Fe, the Texans encountered the Mexican army, who made them surrender. The prisoners were marched over a thousand miles to Mexico City and were put in jail. Some died from cruelty and disease. The ones that survived were released in 1844 to go home. The next year, Texas became a state.

One Student's Initial Textbase, Organized According to the Headings from the Text

1. The Expedition Begins
   a. In 1841, Mirabeau Lamar sent an expedition to Santa Fe.
   b. He wanted to extend a trade path from New York and St. Louis to Santa Fe.
2. Lost in the Canyon
   a. The expedition got lost for weeks in the canyons in West Texas.
   b. Heat and lack of food and water caused their suffering.
3. The Texans Surrender
   a. The Texans encountered the Mexican army right as they got close to Santa Fe.
   b. The Texans surrendered because they were too tired to fight.
4. Imprisoned in Mexico City
   a. The Texans suffered from cruelty and disease.
   b. The ones who survived were released in 1844.

The ARROW strategy has been found to be particularly useful for increasing long-term memory for facts in expository texts. The students referred to in the preceding example earned above-average grades on a test about the Santa Fe expedition.

BRIDGE

BRIDGE utilizes brainstorming, categorization, hierarchical organization, discussion, and self-questioning to facilitate comprehension and long-term recall. Research shows that information that is organized categorically is easier to recall than unorganized information (Albrecht & O'Brien, 1991; Andreassen & Waters, 1989; Hasselhorn, 1995). Headings (or key words) can be especially effective mnemonic devices in hierarchical organization because they can serve as placeholders for more elaborated information. The activation of prior knowledge in existing categories and the efficient addition of new knowledge to previously established categories form the hub of an effortful metacognitive strategy called *BRIDGE*, which is adapted from Garhard (1991).

Suppose that the BRIDGE strategy will be implemented for a social studies lesson on refugee displacement and the United Nations. Assume that the students' task is to learn concepts related to this lesson for an upcoming classroom discussion about worldwide refugee problems and possible solutions.

Step 1

LLD students engage in a brainstorming session to activate background knowledge that can facilitate their understanding of refugee displacement. Key words and phrases (e.g., *war, Bosnia, ethnic fighting, religious differences, lack of food, loss of homes, wandering, suffering*) are listed on an overhead transparency or a chalkboard.

Step 2

The ideas from prior knowledge are categorized into four or five broad headings. For example, the following headings could be delineated:

- causes of refugee problems
- countries with refugee problems
- types of problems refugees experience
- solutions to refugee problems

These headings become superordinates under which subordinate ideas will now be organized.

Step 3

Related ideas from the brainstorming session are organized under the headings. Students are trained to indent the subordinate ideas under the superordinate category as a reminder of the hierarchical structure. For example, subordinate ideas under the superordinate category "types of problems refugees experience" might include the following: lack of food, loss of homes, no jobs, sickness, feelings of worthlessness, and lack of hope.

Step 4

New ideas from the textbook and/or the teacher's lecture about the topic are added to the categories. The focus of this step is the addition of new ideas to join the existing prior knowledge. An example of an additional idea to be added to the causes of refugee displacement might be the desire of one group to dominate another (i.e., domination).

Step 5

LLD adolescents are led through a guided discussion of categorization. The language specialist provides questions related to the major heading (e.g., "Explain some of the causes of refugee problems in today's world"). Students are taught to begin their explanations with a statement about a major heading. This becomes a topic sentence to focus the discussion. For example, "The growing problems of refugees throughout the world and the ensuing resettlement issues can generally be traced to similar causes." Next, students elaborate by expressing ideas from the list of subordinate items related to the topic sentence. In this example, they may add to the discussion with statements like, "Religious conflicts and ethnic fighting cause wars. People who leave their homes to escape the war become refugees."

Step 6

Finally, adolescents are trained in self-questioning. This self-questioning procedure continues to emphasize the utilization of hierarchical structure as adolescents move toward greater independence in preparing for class discussions. However, self-questioning also can be applied to their preparation for examinations and writing assignments. These are the questions adolescents should ask themselves:

- Have I identified the major headings related to the topic?
- Did I select and organize the facts appropriately for each heading?
- Have I remembered to eliminate trivial information from related facts?
- Have I planned transitional phrases that will link successive categories? (Garhard, 1991)

Step 7

This is the recall step in the BRIDGE strategy. After an interval of several days or weeks, the language specialist assesses the adolescent's efficiency in utilizing categorization for recall. In one recall technique, the language specialist provides subordinate ideas and requests students to provide major headings. Students are expected to utilize categorization to facilitate recall. A second recall technique involves giving students headings (categories) and asking them to assemble the related items (Garhard, 1991). The BRIDGE strategy provides a way to activate prior knowledge and mesh new knowledge with existing categories to facilitate efficient recall.

THE RELUCTANT STRATEGY USER

Just as an umbrella is a useless tool in rain until it is opened up as a protective covering, an effortful strategy is useless until it is utilized successfully in appropriate contexts. Language specialists need to determine those factors that affect strategy selection and use by LLD students. Keep in mind that a developmental milestone in adolescence is the movement to independence. The specialist who neglects to plan how to sell adolescents on the importance of using a strategy may be wasting much of the valuable time spent in strategy teaching.

Why might an LLD adolescent underutilize or neglect to implement a learned strategy? Siegler and Shipley's (1995) suggestions about the selection or nonselection of known mathematical strategies are applied here to adolescent LLD students:

- *The LLD adolescent may fail to be convinced of a strategy's utility in problem solving.* Strategy practice during intervention sessions may not be connected to the planning and problem-solving requirements of the regular curriculum. The language specialist should help LLD adolescents connect strategies to eventual outcomes. Many adolescents may be hardened by past failures. The extra effort taken to identify problems in the youths' school, home, or work life and to carefully select metacognitive and retrieval strategies to teach will lead to better results.

- *The LLD adolescent may believe the extra effort that a deliberate metacognitive strategy requires diminishes the strategy's usefulness.* Strategy selection is often evaluated for speed of implementation. Adolescents may cast aside a useful strategy because it fails to meet their personal criterion of "economy of effort." In other words, adolescents will not use strategies that they find too lengthy or cumbersome. The language specialist who has a thorough knowledge of the LLD adolescent's interests, goals, and future plans will be better able to identify motivators to offset the extra effort metacognitive strategies initially require. The language specialist can consider such motivational forces as these: Will utilizing known metacognitive strategies aid in keeping the LLD adolescent on his or her school sports team because the youth's grades will improve? Will the extra time to utilize strategies result in positive feedback from teachers and parents? Will the strategy improve his or her interaction and reputation among peers? Will the strategy salvage the LLD youth's poor performance in a class that is needed to meet graduation requirements? Knowledge about the motivators in an adolescent's life can be used in convincing students that the extra effort a strategy may require will produce desirable outcomes toward one or more of the LLD adolescent's personal goals.
- *The LLD adolescent may not equate effective strategy implementation with success in problem solving.* This point is related to convincing the adolescent of a connection between strategy utilization and desired outcomes. An improved grade on a science project that is the direct result of applying metacognitive strategies may still be thought of as "luck." Students' unwillingness to trust that their efforts could bring success may be rooted in a history of repeated failures. The language specialist must overcome the adolescent's belief in luck by having the student successfully utilize a known effortful metacognitive strategy a sufficient number of times to eliminate the belief in luck as the sole possibility of strategy success.

BECOMING STRATEGIC

Once students know two or three learning strategies, they need to learn how to act strategically. That is, students must realize how to select and modify the strategies they know to meet the demands of various situations. For example, the language specialist's role could involve moving adolescents toward recognizing when the ARROW or BRIDGE metacognitive strategies should be applied. Strategic training can incorporate a task analysis wherein adolescents appropriate a metastrategy. They can learn to ask questions such as these: "What exactly must I accomplish to be successful with this task?" "Which steps in the strategies I know might work efficiently and accurately in this context?"

Being strategic involves a planned effort specifically generated for a particular goal. It can be compared to the dart thrower who assumes a certain stance and posture in the planned effort to hit the bull's-eye or the golfer's strategic selection of a particular club and utilization of a certain swing to reach the green. As applied to academic situations, adolescents who need to pass a test on information presented in an expository text might decide to use some or all of the steps in the ARROW strategy. Those who are preparing for class discussions, regardless of the topic, might select the BRIDGE strategy.

Strategic action implies recognizing new problems that may have underlying similarities to previously solved problems. Consider an LLD adolescent with a goal of getting a part-time job. One of his obstacles might be improving his academic performance so that his parents will allow him to search for a job. Suppose that this student has a strong academic standing in his drafting class, yet he is barely passing algebra and social studies. In this case, the goal is improved grades in algebra and social studies, and the obstacle is the student's poor performance on the last two assignments and/or examinations in both classes.

Each class concerns different content. The student's job is to determine whether there is any strategy from drafting class that can be applied to algebra class and social studies class. Assume that the student has met regularly with his drafting instructor for review and/or demonstration of projects. The student can be trained to ask the question, "Wouldn't that same strategy be applicable to the algebra and social studies classes as a step toward the goal of improved grades?" Although each class covers different material, the plan to reach a desired outcome in an academic environment has a similar underlying structure—get explanation, clarification, and/or demonstration of class material from the instructor. This is strategic action in operation.

Crisafi and Brown (1986) offer several ways that a language specialist can scaffold an LLD adolescent toward strategic action. These include providing hints, discussion and reflection, and allowing the student to teach. All three methods can be socially mediated as the language specialist frames learning within interactions that provide opportunities to discover desired knowledge. A hint is a statement to the LLD adolescent that the next problem will be "like the one we just did." This is a deliberate push by the language specialist to effect knowledge transfer and problem solving. During discussion, the language specialist may present a problem and request that the LLD adolescent compare the new problem to a previously solved problem. Finally, knowledge is often unlocked as one stretches to explain, clarify, and/or demonstrate to someone else. The third step, then, encourages the language specialist to afford the LLD adolescent opportunities to teach strategic action to someone else. The inclusion of peer teaching in the metacognitive process taps an essential ingredient of adolescent life: interaction with one's friends. If metacognitive strategies can gain some utility in the LLD adolescent's daily interactions, there will be opportunities for known strategies to receive more frequent application. The time spent in gaining an in-depth understanding of the adolescent and his or her goals will benefit numerous aspects of the intervention process.

COST AND BENEFIT ANALYSIS

Just as there is variation in processing capacities in individuals with language impairments (e.g., Lahey & Bloom, 1994; Weismer, 1995), there is a good deal of variability in the way LLD adolescents respond to the strategy selection process. Despite this inherent variability, a cost and benefit analysis of performance and use of effortful strategies may play an important role in self-regulating the use of effortful strategies.

Economy of effort

Economy of effort is operative in many aspects of the speech production process, so it is not surprising to have it raised in the strategy selection process. Strategies that require several steps take longer, so their outcomes need to be relevant and easily perceived if they are going to be used in independent learning situations. Economy of effort has its benefits, but it can be quite costly if critical steps are omitted, resulting in failed solutions or outcomes. Clinicians and adolescents need to discuss the costs and benefits of economy of effort and its link to goal achievement. Goal clarification and assessment of the costs and benefits of speed in accessing knowledge versus accuracy in accessing knowledge often need to be reviewed repeatedly. Students are much more likely to utilize a time-intensive metacognitive strategy when it helps them achieve their personal, academic, or career goals.

Strategy novelty and accuracy

Siegler and Shipley (1995) have emphasized the short life of metacognitive strategies that fail to result in desired solutions. The language specialist needs to reduce utilization deficiencies, or only the most frequently used strategies will stay on the LLD adolescent's mental shelf. If the deliberate and automatic strategies that students are currently using result in passing grades or at least marginally satisfying peer interactions, why should they select new, less economic strategies? Again, knowledge of the adolescents' personal goals, their abilities, and the academic and personal problems they face is critical to effective instruction. Students need to be shown that better outcomes are worth the extra effort of applying a new effortful strategy rather than resorting to an older, well-rehearsed, automatic strategy that may not apply to the learning contexts that are typical of middle school and high school courses.

•   •   •

Adolescents who cannot make the transition to self-regulated learning during the middle school and high school years are at serious risk for academic, vocational, and social failure. Many of these students need to learn how to understand and remember information that is contained in outside reading assignments. Presented here were two effortful metacognitive strategies, ARROW and BRIDGE, that can be used to facilitate self-regulated learning and long-term retention of information. Students who master effortful strategies such as these will have made important steps toward achieving academic success.

Knowing how to follow the steps in an effortful strategy should not be the end goal of any intervention program with LLD adolescents. Students need to know how to act strategically: to apply those strategies that will result in the most success with the least amount of effort. To this end, a metastrategy helps students find similarities in the underlying goal structures in various problems. When students recognize that a given problem shares similar attributes with problems they already know how to solve, they will be well on the way to strategic behavior.

REFERENCES

Albrecht, J.E., & O'Brien, E.J. (1991). Effects of centrality on retrieval of text-based concepts. *Journal of Experimental Psychology: Learning, Memory, and Cognition, 17,* 932–939.

Anderson, R.C. (1994). Role of the reader's schema in comprehension, learning, and memory. In R.B. Ruddell, M.R. Ruddell, & H. Singer (Eds.), *Theoretical models and processes of reading* (4th ed., pp. 469–482). Newark, DE: International Reading Association.

Anderson, R.C., & Pichert, J.W. (1978). Recall of previously unrecallable information following a shift in perspective. *Journal of Verbal Learning and Verbal Behavior, 17,* 1–12.

Andreassen, C., & Waters, H.S. (1989). Organization during study: Relationships between metamemory, strategy use, and performance. *Journal of Educational Psychology, 81,* 170–191.

Bjorklund, D.F., & Coyle, T.R. (1995). Utilization deficiencies in the development of memory strategies. In F.E. Weinert & W. Schneider (Eds.), *Memory performance and competencies: Issues in growth and development* (pp. 161–180). Mahwah, NJ: Lawrence Erlbaum Associates.

Brown, A. (1989). Analogical learning and transfer: What develops? In S. Vosniadou & A. Ortony (Eds.), *Similarity and analogical reasoning* (pp. 369–412). Cambridge, England: Cambridge University Press.

Carrell, P. (1992). Awareness of text structure: Effects on recall. *Language Learning, 42,* 1–20.

Ceci, S.J., Lea, S.E., & Ringstrom, M.D. (1980). Coding processes in normal and learning-disabled children: Evidence for modality-specific pathways to the cognitive system. *Journal of Experimental Psychology: Human Learning and Memory, 6,* 785–797.

Cooney, J.R., & Swanson, H.L. (1987). Memory and learning disabilities: An overview. In H.L. Swanson (Ed.), *Memory and learning disabilities* (pp. 1–40). Greenwich, CT: JAJ Press.

Crisafi, M., & Brown, A. (1986). Analogical transfer in very young children: Combining two separately learned solutions to reach goal. *Child Development, 57,* 953–968.

Dallago, M.L., & Moeley, B.E. (1980). Free recall in boys of normal and poor reading levels as a function of task manipulations. *Journal of Experimental Child Psychology*, *30*, 62–78.

Flavell, J.H. (1985). *Cognitive development* (2nd ed.). Englewood Cliffs, NJ: Prentice Hall.

Foos, P.W. (1992). Constructing schemata while reading simple stories. *Journal of General Psychology*, *119*, 419–425.

Garhard, C. (1991). *Assessment of conceptual organization (ACO): Improving writing, thinking, and reading skills*. Philadelphia: Research for Better Schools.

Graham, S., MacArthur, C., Schwartz, S., & Voth, T. (1992). Improving the compositions of students with learning disabilities using a strategy involving product and process goal setting. *Exceptional Children*, *58*, 322–335.

Hasselhorn, M. (1995). Beyond production deficiency and utilization inefficiency: Mechanisms of the emergence of strategic categorization in episodic memory tasks. In F.E. Weinert & W. Schneider (Eds.), *Memory performance and competencies: Issues in growth and development* (pp. 141–160). Mahwah, NJ: Lawrence Erlbaum Associates.

Jacoby, L.L., Levy, B.A., & Steinbach, K. (1992). Episodic transfer and automaticity: Integration of data-driven and conceptually-driven processing in rereading. *Journal of Experimental Psychology: Learning, Memory, and Cognition*, *18*, 15–24.

Kail, R., & Leonard, L. (1986). Word-finding abilities in language-impaired children. *ASHA Monographs*, *25*, 1–39.

Lahey, M., & Bloom, L. (1994). Variability and language learning disabilities. In G. Wallach & K. Butler (Eds.), *Language learning disabilities in school-age children and adolescents* (pp. 354–372). Needham Heights, MA: Allyn & Bacon.

Levy, B.A., Di Persio, R., & Hollingshead, A. (1992). Fluent rereading: Repetition, automaticity, and discrepancy. *Journal of Experimental Psychology*, *18*, 957–971.

McDaniel, M.A., Einstein, G.O., & Waddill, P.J. (1990). Material-appropriate processing: Implications for remediating recall deficits in students with learning disabilities. *Learning Disabilities Quarterly*, *13*, 258–268.

McKeown, M.G., Beck, I.L., Sinatra, G.M., & Loxterman, J.A. (1992). The contribution of prior knowledge and coherent text to comprehension. *Reading Research Quarterly*, *27*, 78–93.

Palinscar, A., & Brown, A. (1984). Reciprocal teaching of comprehension-fostering and comprehension-monitoring activities. *Cognition and Instruction*, *1*, 117–175.

Pressley, M., & Harris, K. (1990). What we really know about strategy instruction. *Education Leadership*, *48*(1), 31–34.

Sawyer, R., Graham, S., & Harris, K.R. (1992). Direct teaching, strategy instruction, and strategy instruction with explicit self-regulation: Effects on learning disabled students' compositions and self-efficacy. *Journal of Educational Psychology*, *84*, 340–352.

Schmalhofer, F. (1995). The acquisition of knowledge from text and example situations: An extension to the construction-integration model. In C.A. Weaver, S. Mannes, & C.R. Fletcher (Eds.), *Discourse comprehension: Essays in honor of Walter Kintsch* (pp. 257–283). Hillsdale, NJ: Lawrence Erlbaum Associates.

Siegler, R., & Shipley, C. (1995). Variation, selection and cognitive change. In T. Simon & G. Halford (Eds.), *Developing cognitive competence* (pp. 31–76). Hillsdale, NJ: Lawrence Erlbaum Associates.

Siegler, R., & Shrager, J. (1984). Strategy choices in addition and subtraction: How do children know what to do? In C. Sophian (Ed.), *Origins of cognitive skills* (pp. 229–293). Hillsdale, NJ: Lawrence Erlbaum Associates.

Swanson, H.L. (1986). Learning disabled readers' verbal coding difficulties: A problem of storage or retrieval? *Learning Disabilities Research, 1*, 73–82.

Swanson, H.L., Reffel, J., & Trahan, M. (1991). Naturalistic memory in learning-disabled and skilled readers. *Journal of Abnormal Child Psychology, 19*, 117–147.

van Dijk, T., & Kintsch, W. (1983). *Strategies of discourse comprehension*. Orlando, FL: Academic Press.

Wallach, G.P., & Miller, L. (1988). *Language intervention and academic success*. Boston: College-Hill.

Weismer, S.E. (1995). Capacity limitations in working memory: The impact of lexical and morphological learning by children with language impairment. *Topics in Language Disorders, 17*(1), 33–44.

10

Functional Treatment Approaches to Memory Impairment Following Brain Injury

Judith Hutchinson and Thomas P. Marquardt

Treatment of cognitive disorders resulting from brain injury must extend beyond intervention strategies focusing on deficit reduction to embrace paradigms centering on disability reduction. Disability-oriented approaches emphasize rehearsal and encoding strategies and the use of memory aids. Following consideration of cognitive memory deficits in brain injury, specific strategies will be considered that focus on disability reduction in individuals with brain injury.

CLINICAL FEATURES OF MEMORY IMPAIRMENT

Results from surveys of patients and family members (Brooks, 1984; Mateer, Sohlberg, & Crineon, 1987; McKinlay, Brooks, Martinage, & Marshall, 1981) concur with many clinicians' observations that one of the most frequent and persistent cognitive impairments following brain injury is memory disturbance. Long after most physical disabilities have reached stabilization or recovery, lingering memory problems prevent many survivors of brain injury from returning to active employment, independent living, or full social lives. One feature of memory changes related to brain injury that is often particularly troubling to patients and family members is the phenomenon of differential memory abilities, sometimes interpreted by frustrated families as a "selective" memory impairment. The demonstration of preserved memory for previously learned information and pro-

Top Lang Disord 1997;18(1):45–57
© 1997 Aspen Publishers, Inc.

cesses, contrasting sharply with significant difficulty learning or remembering new or recent information, presents a striking dichotomy, frequently interpreted in lay language as a "short-term memory problem." This terminological (and conceptual) error can lead to confusion when patients and families encounter professional literature using this term, as well as when clinicians communicate on different levels of understanding of memory concepts. The clinician can assist the family—and other clinicians less familiar with memory function and terminology—by striving to provide and use less problematic language for discussing memory. To assist in that effort, memory terminology, as well as models for classification and description of memory function, are presented. The authors offer a descriptive scaffolding for memory to serve as the framework for discussion of intervention strategies.

MEMORY TERMINOLOGY, CONCEPTS, AND MODELING

One simple system for description and modeling of memory is in terms of length of storage of information. The subsystems of this model are labeled *sensory, short-term,* and *long-term memory.*

Sensory memory is a large-capacity, short-term store of information specific to a sensory modality. The two forms of sensory memory most fully described, and most relevant to communication, are (1) visual, or *iconic,* memory and (2) auditory, or *echoic,* memory. A perceived stimulus is retained in sensory memory for a matter of milliseconds before fading. The integrity of this stage of memory input is crucial to longer term storage, and an impairment at this level may invalidate attempts to rehabilitate memory at other levels. While a relevant factor in the overall memory impairments of most patients with brain injury, and sometimes explicitly addressed in rehabilitation (Parenté & Anderson-Parenté, 1991), sensory memory is not usually a primary route for treatment of memory problems.

Short-term memory (*STM*) is more appropriately referred to as *immediate* memory, reflecting its denotation of a limited-capacity, short-term store. In everyday activity, it is the memory for events that just happened, such as a phone number read from the directory and remembered long enough to dial. A number (or other information) is "kept" in STM only a few seconds unless it is repeated or intentionally memorized. The process of keeping a memory trace active in memory is termed *rehearsal*; this is demonstrated when one repeats the number until able to dial it and discard it from memory, without future retention of the number. While the term *STM* implies a "place" for storage of information, the term and concept of *working memory* (*WM*; Baddeley & Hitch, 1974) more accurately captures the dynamic quality of the temporary memory store used in information processing. WM refers to STM when it is being used to solve a problem or perform a task (Cowan, 1996, Chapter 1). Impairment in STM or WM presents a "bottleneck," preventing the addition of new information to long-term storage.

Long-term memory (*LTM*) refers to a large-capacity, long-term store of information, scripts, procedures, rules, and so forth. The capacity is virtually infinite, as is the length of time information can be retained in LTM. In everyday activity, this is the memory demonstrated when one recalls a name hours after meeting someone, remembers having a conversation with a friend the day before, or remembers vocabulary learned as a child. Notice that this concept includes all information stored for more than a few seconds, whether the memory is acquired recently or long ago, after onset of a brain injury or before. LTM is thus the form of memory most crucial for acquisition and retention of new information as well as access to all previously learned information. LTM is also the domain of the lexicon and other linguistic information and, thus, crucial to communication. Finally, the integrity of access to LTM is particularly necessary to the young survivor of brain injury who is engaged in academic or vocational training.

Some dissociations in memory function often observed by families and clinicians reflect important differentiations of memory content and operation, usually described in terms of dichotomies or contrasting pairs.

Patients and families have long observed that which research has clearly demonstrated to be a distinction in types of memory access and retrieval. *Declarative memory*, often equated with *explicit,* or *conscious,* memory, is the conscious recollection of information. *Nondeclarative memory*, also termed *implicit,* or *unconscious,* memory, refers to information that can be demonstrated to be stored and accessed but without conscious knowledge of the memory process. Declarative memory is often impaired with brain injury; nondeclarative memory is rarely impaired (Gabrieli, McGlinchey-Berroth, Carrillo, Cermak, & Disterhoft, 1995). The relative preservation of nondeclarative memory is demonstrated by preserved motor learning, stimulus association learning, and, of particular relevance to communication function, the effect of *priming*. Priming is enhanced retrieval of information, following a previous presentation of the information, without conscious knowledge of the memory (Glisky & Schacter, 1987). Retained priming effects, despite impaired declarative recall ability, permit the use of cuing strategies in intervention with many patients. In addition to priming, *procedural memory*—skill-based, stimulus-response learning, particularly of motor skills—is usually preserved relative to explicit memory skills (Knowlton, Mangels, & Squire, 1996). Self-awareness of procedural skills competence is normally low without additional declarative coding of the information, a fact consistent with the usually poor self-knowledge and performance-prediction abilities of patients with brain injury.

Declarative memory includes *semantic memory*, or context-independent memory for factual information, without necessarily having declarative knowledge of where the information was acquired. *Episodic memory*, or context-dependent memory for specific events, includes autobiographical information, while *lexical memory* (often considered a form of semantic memory) includes knowledge of phonetic, orthographic, and morphological information about lexical items. Semantic and lexical memory may be differentially impaired in brain injury.

Memory, once thought to be a unitary process, has been demonstrated to be divisible into dissociable subsystems. Such dissociation is apparent experimentally as well as in cases of brain injury, with relative preservation of nondeclarative forms of memory and procedural learning, even in a context of significantly impaired declarative memory function. Because of the vulnerability of the declarative memory system to impairment from brain injury, and the impact of such impairment on rehabilitation, the focus of this chapter is on the declarative memory systems.

NEUROANATOMICAL SUBSTRATE FOR MEMORY

Evidence from neuropathology, as well as from neuroimaging studies of normal memory behavior, indicates involvement of medial temporal, diencephalic, and frontal areas in normal declarative memory processes. The hippocampus, amygdala, and adjacent related medial temporal areas are involved in STM operations. In particular, the hippocampus is strongly implicated in transferal of potentially transient STM information into a more permanent form in the neocortex (Zasler, 1991). The existence of temporally graded retrograde amnesia phenomena, that is, more difficulty recalling recent than remote retrograde information, suggests a gradual consolidation process, with diminishing importance of the medial temporal structures and increased neocortical involvement as LTM information is stored (Rempel-Clower, Zola, Squire, & Amaral, 1996; Squire & Alvarez, 1995). Positron emission tomography (PET) studies support the idea that interruption of the postencoding consolidation process by traumatic brain injury may result in temporally graded retrograde amnesia (Mattiolli et al., 1996).

The neuroanatomical correlates of retrieval from LTM have been described through case studies and PET research. Inferolateral frontal and anterolateral temporal cortical areas—distinct from the medial temporal and diencephalic regions involved in new memory formation—appear to be associated with the retrieval process (Markowitsch, 1995). Disconnection of neocortical memory engram loci from the frontal-temporal retrieval system (bidirectionally connected by the uncinate fascicle) may result in retrieval impairments despite evidence of preserved storage of information. Within this frontal-temporal memory retrieval system, there may be distinct functions associated with the frontal and temporal areas. For example, frontally based memory operations correspond with other functions usually associated with the frontal lobes, such as control, supervision, sequencing, and organization, while temporal operations correspond with temporal-lobe connections to posterior cortical centers and the primary storage loci of the memory engrams (Markowitsch, 1995).

Material-specific hemispheric specialization appears to apply to some but not all aspects of memory function. "Rehabilitation folklore" tends to assume the existence of independent, completely dissociable verbal and nonverbal memory systems, while, in fact, differences in memory function related to *hemisphericity* of brain damage most closely correlate with integrity of the sensory, perceptual, and analytical systems that are specific to an individual's initial processing and demonstration of successful retrieval of linguistic, spatial, or other types of material. Hemispheric asymmetries are evident, however, in PET studies contrasting retrieval of episodic versus semantic information from LTM, with right hemisphere specialization for episodic memory function and left hemisphere for semantic memory (Markowitsch, 1995).

Corresponding to current memory systems models demonstrating dissociable subsystems and memory types, the neuroanatomical substrate for memory function also demonstrates multiple, dissociable systems for memory acquisition and access. The medial temporal and diencephalic systems are involved in memory acquisition and consolidation, while a frontal-temporal system is involved in retrieval from LTM. In cases of individuals with brain injury, any or all of these systems may be vulnerable to damage; the frontal and temporal poles (retrieval system) are particularly vulnerable to primary injury, as are the medial temporal area and diencephalon (encoding/consolidation system), and multiple cortical and subcortical areas, especially in the frontal lobes (executive functions affecting memory), may be damaged with resulting indirect effects on memory abilities.

Structures of the frontal and temporal lobes are vulnerable to brain injury at the skull-brain interface, including contusions of the cortical surface but particularly the hippocampus and other more medial limbic structures of the temporal lobe (Bigler, 1990). The primary trauma effects are the result of diffuse, nonspecific neuronal shear-strain effects (Adams, Graham, & Gennarelli, 1985) upon which superimposed focal lesions may be found. These diffuse axonal injuries are characterized by torn axonal fibers, glial cell damage, and neuronal degeneration distal from the location of shearing (Bigler, 1990). The primary damage lies in deep white fiber pathways and the brain stem. When coupled with altered vascular dynamics, anoxia with ischemic necrosis of tissue, structural compression and herniation of brain tissue due to edema, and hemorrhage, significant deficits in memory are expected (Uzzell, Obrist, Dolinskas, & Langfitt, 1986).

ASSESSMENT OF MEMORY FUNCTION

Appropriate rehabilitation of memory-related cognitive deficits requires thorough assessment of the individual's memory. However, the details of that process are not agreed upon universally. Traditional neuropsychological measures permit delineating differential areas of impairment, confirming the presence of primary memory impairment, and identifying indirect factors affecting memory function. Standardized neuropsychological assessment is particularly useful for (1) patient education and awareness training, (2) documentation of need for rehabilitation services, and (3) decision making with regard to academic and vocational placements. In addition, thorough assessment of underlying linguistic abilities, via conventional language testing, provides standard measures of integrity of language at the impairment level of analysis. Areas to include in assessment reflect the dissociations in memory systems at the functional and neuroanatomical levels. For excellent comprehensive guides to assessment of memory, particularly with respect to traumatic brain injury, see Harrell,

Parenté, Bellingrath, and Lisicia (1992); Lezak (1995); and Parenté and Herrmann (1996).

Clinicians are increasingly aware of the problem of "ecological validity" of any cognitive assessment measure; for an excellent discussion of this issue, see Acker (1990). Particularly with regard to communication-related memory function, effective assessment and treatment are dependent on the patient's demonstration of impairment effects appearing at the level of disability, that is, the inability to perform some functional activity. For treatment planning, patient/family education, and progress/outcome measurement, valid functional measures must be quantified. Unfortunately, formal instruments for assessment of functional abilities are limited, difficult to standardize, and sometimes controversial. The Rivermead Behavioral Memory Test (Wilson, Cockburn, Baddeley, & Hiorns, 1989) was designed as a functional memory test battery and includes test probes simulating "real-life" memory situations, such as remembering to deliver a message, recalling a route, and remembering the name of a "new" person when cued with that person's picture.

In addition, questionnaires and rating scales are recommended in order to quantify information from patients, family members, and rehabilitation staff about patients' everyday memory behavior. Available materials include the Present Functioning Questionnaire (Tuokko & Crockett, 1991), Prospective Memory Process Training Memory Questionnaire (Mateer et al., 1987), Multimodal Inventory of Cognitive Status (Parenté & Herrmann, 1996), Cognitive Failures Questionnaire (Broadbent, Cooper, Fitzgerald, & Parkes, 1982), Everyday Memory Questionnaire (Sunderland, Harris, & Gleave, 1984), Brief Cognitive Rating Scale (Reisberg & Ferris, 1982), and more general functional rating scales such as the Instrumental Activities of Daily Living Scale (Lawton & Brody, 1969; Tuokko & Crockett, 1991). Often, the most effective memory rehabilitation approaches involve utilization of external memory aids in compensation for, rather than restoration of, memory impairment. Successful use of compensatory aids should be evaluated on assessment measures but may not be if standard neuropsychological assessment measures are used exclusively. Recommended approaches to assessment of everyday memory and use of compensatory aids should include assessment of the following:

- orientation with external aids available (clock, signs, notebook, schedule, calendar, etc.)

- evaluation of knowledge of and demonstrated proficiency in use of external aids such as organizers or notebooks
- evaluation of effective/appropriate external aid use in functional activities such as time management/getting to therapies on one's own, self-management of medication, an independent exercise program, and participation in social activities including phone use
- assessment of initiation and appropriate use of external aids in prospective memory activities

REHABILITATION OF MEMORY

Much of the controversy about rehabilitation of memory—and, in fact, about cognitive rehabilitation in general—involves differences in interpretation of the concept of rehabilitation. Efficacy of treatment depends on which approach, or combination of approaches, is used. Wilson (1987) provides a useful summary of theories of recovery and rehabilitation. She concludes that restorative approaches (stimulation, neural regeneration, anatomical reorganization) are the least likely to be primary factors in recovery, while other methods (including environmental cuing and aids, supportive therapy, and utilization of internal strategies such as mnemonics) can significantly improve functional performance. Prigatano (1990) emphasizes the importance of a "realistic" approach to memory rehabilitation, with a focus on patient education and awareness and on compensatory versus restorative treatment. Efficacy of individual rehabilitation programs depends on the degree of utilization of this broader approach to rehabilitation.

Most rehabilitation clinicians receive little or no explicit training in treatment of memory impairments but frequently express a need for treatment methods appropriate to the brain-injured population and find themselves uncomfortably improvising or using memory-improvement routines designed for the non–brain-damaged population. A conceptual framework is useful in discussion of treatment approaches to any cognitive impairment. A framework can help clarify the method appropriate to the specific population under consideration. Parenté and Herrmann (1996) describe categories of intervention in terms of (1) active variables (operations affecting the content of the information in the cognitive system), (2) passive variables (factors affecting the patient's readiness or inclination, including physiological and emotional factors), and (3) support variables (environmental factors including prosthetic devices).

A variation of this framework (Hutchinson, 1993) applies well to memory impairment and will be used to discuss efficacy, methodology, and appropriate populations for a variety of memory treatment methods. The first few types of intervention described require minimal patient initiation or active participation; later types require explicit training, practice, and assessment of generalization.

Medical and pharmacological intervention

Zasler (1991) reviews pharmacological approaches to modification of cognitive function, including utilization of medications potentially facilitating cognition (hypothalamic and pituitary neuropeptides, cholinergic agonists, catecholaminergic agonists, nootropics, vasoactive agents) and minimization of use of medications potentially interfering with cognition (catecholaminergic antagonists, gabaminergic agonists, and cholinergic antagonists). Although, as he indicates, there is no "magic bullet" for cognitive enhancement, the impact of pharmacological factors can be significant in overall function and prognosis. In addition, medical management of seizures, edema, and other acute conditions affecting neurological integrity are obviously crucial factors in rehabilitation potential and should be addressed during cognitive rehabilitation.

Peripheral factors

This approach includes remediation of any problems that may indirectly interfere with the patient's ability to receive sensory information, attend and concentrate, and utilize external aids. Remediation at this level demands little or no participation by, or training of, the patient. Examples of peripheral factors remediation approaches include correction of impaired vision and audition; use of orthotics, such as eye patches to temporarily relieve diplopia; improved nutrition and hydration; adjustment of medications indirectly affecting attention and memory; relief of pain by positioning, relaxation, or medication; and control of rest and sleep pattern through scheduling and medication.

Environmental management

This approach also requires little patient participation but can provide significant remediation of memory impairments. Examples of environmental remediation include provision of labeled receptacles for personal items (such as keys, glasses, dentures), signs on cabinets indicating contents, and reminder signs to cue activities or needs (such as medications). The integrity of language function must be considered in determining appropriate types of reminders.

Family/caregiver education and training

Similar in effect to environmental management, this approach requires little patient participation or training but provides increased potential for independence through improved support from the social environment. Primary areas for caregiver education include thorough explanation of the patient's memory abilities, clarification of any confusion about "selective" memory problems, explanation and demonstration of appropriate cuing and supervision methods, and suggestions for environmental structure.

Awareness and adjustment training

Patient awareness of deficit has been demonstrated to be a significant factor in rehabilitation potential. Crosson et al. (1989) describe different levels of awareness:

- *Intellectual awareness* is the ability to understand and verbalize deficit knowledge.
- *Compensatory awareness* is the slightly more advanced ability to identify errors and correct them.
- *Anticipatory awareness* is the demonstrated ability to prepare for and prevent potential problems resulting from cognitive impairments.

The memory-impaired patient must be assessed for current level of awareness and presented with educational and counseling support appropriate to that level in order that awareness be gradually increased. Group therapy approaches are particularly effective in providing peer feedback and improving insight into deficits. Video feedback is also frequently employed for awareness training, including treatment to facilitate communication in context, message repair, and cohesiveness of narrative (Ehrlich & Sipes, 1985).

Restorative and process-specific approaches

Many popular approaches to memory improvement, including those designed for the non–brain-injured population, are based on an assumption that repetitive use, practice, and placement of increased demands on a cognitive system will result in neurological adaptation and recovery. General "stimulation" approaches have been found to have minimal and only generalized effects on overall cognitive function. However, narrowly focused direct retraining of cognitive processes through hierarchically arranged treatment (the process approach described and utilized by Bracy [1986] and Sohlberg and Mateer [1987]) has been shown to be effective in the rehabilitation of some types of linguistic and cognitive impairments. Process-specific training has been used most effectively in attention training and probably least effectively in memory training. The crucial role of attention in memory function—in encoding, rehearsal, consolidation, and retrieval processes—indicates the utility of providing attention-process training as part of a memory rehabilitation program. However, repetitive practice in memorization and frequent demands to remember material, although still frequently observed in rehabilitation settings, have not been shown to be useful in memory improvement and, in fact, are likely to be detrimental to the therapy process (Prigatano et al., 1984).

Personal compensatory strategy training

In contrast to restorative approaches, compensatory strategy training emphasizes conscious utilization of cognitive facilitation techniques. "Personal" compensatory strategies (i.e., internal to the patient) include increasing conscious attention, utilizing rehearsal techniques, and operating on the specific content material to enhance its encoding and subsequent retrieval.

Rehearsal training is less familiar to most rehabilitation therapists than are other types of personal compensatory strategies for memory training. Rehearsal is the process of repetition of information in WM in order to enhance its consolidation into LTM. This is, to some extent, an automatic, unconscious process in normal function. However, automaticity of processing is impaired in brain injury. Therefore, rehearsal training is based on the premise that brain-injured patients require explicit, conscious rehearsal of information in order to effect its consolidation. Fortunately, it has been demonstrated to be effective and easily taught to patients with brain injury. Parenté and Anderson-Parenté (1991) introduced the strategy to patients by first asking them to memorize information before being shown the strategy, then repeating the same activity with forced rehearsal of the material. The rehearsal results in immediate improvement in easily compared scores, thus engaging the patient in further training of the method. Then, rehearsal is practiced in a variety of settings to improve its automaticity and tap into procedural learning abilities. While this strategy requires training in identifying the material to be memorized and conscious use of a strategy to effect the memorization, it does not demand that patients develop explicit mnemonics or other content-based methods. Elements of personal compensatory strategy are clearly evident in the functional-integrative and compensatory training described by Ylvisaker and Holland (1985) and Hartley (1995).

Familiar traditional examples of content-oriented strategies are use of visual imagery or of first-letter reminders to recall information. Categories of these types of strategies are described by Parenté and Herrmann (1996):

- perceptual grouping (e.g., clustering numbers in a phone number)
- organization (e.g., categorizing items in a grocery list)
- mediation (e.g., self-questioning, use of mnemonics)
- mental imagery (e.g., visualizing items together, as in linking in a story format)
- association (e.g., learning new names by linking to a facial feature)

Parenté, Twum, and Zoltan (1994) described the efficacy of such "learning instruction," noting improved performance in specific items learned, such as directions or names. Visual imagery techniques have been demonstrated to help patients learn paired associates and verbal lists. However, extended use of personal strategies is rarely independently initiated by patients, requires considerable executive and reasoning functions, and often demands good verbal-linguistic ability (e.g., in developing mnemonics). Thus, while therapists can assist patients in learning specific information, most patients do not demonstrate significant independent use of strategies to improve their recall (Richardson, 1995).

Domain-specific training

Glisky and Schacter (1987) investigated the use of preserved learning abilities—evidenced by priming effects—in acquisition of specific knowledge and procedures. Patients who were not able to recall previous training trials still were able to demonstrate learning of procedures and terminology, through the "vanishing cues" approach. This approach requires that the therapist provide full cuing initially, while fading cues on subsequent trials. Training in the use of external memory aids is usually approached as a specialized form of domain-specific training; that is, the patient is trained to use a specific system, utilizing priming and procedural learning ability. Correct use of adaptive devices and physical mobility aids, the learning of routes and schedules, and self-administration of exercise programs have all been effectively taught through the domain-specific approach. Generalization of such domain-specific training to other knowledge and situations is predictably limited. Since this approach is intended to provide a route for acquisition of specific knowledge, repeated training programs will be required for new domains of knowledge or skill.

The TRACES protocol (Hutchinson & Watkins, 1994), developed with significant input from a brain-injury survivor, incorporates the positive qualities of external cuing strategies into realistic solutions to everyday memory problems. Negative associations with cuing systems are minimized. In this system, the patient learns to associate increasingly abstract reminders with specific activities to be performed. The critical features of this approach are overcoming automaticity, providing salient attention-getting cues to interrupt routines; providing adequate specificity to cue the appropriate activity; and, most important to many individuals with brain injury, adjusting the system to meet the psychosocial needs of the user.

External compensatory aid training

External aid training requires patient participation and investment in the process, but the use of external memory devices is familiar to the general public and does not tend to be threatening or confusing to the patient. Ideally, external aids already in use by the patient are incorporated into the overall assistive device planning. In addition, alternative devices and systems should be investigated, in collaboration with the patient, if other cognitive or physical factors preclude full use of existing systems or if those systems are inadequate. Harrell et al. (1992) and Parenté and Herrmann (1996) provide detailed descriptions of a wide variety of available external aid devices.

The most popular and well-known method is the use of the "memory notebook," usually an individually designed system for organizing personal and scheduling information. Examples of notebook contents include the following:

- autobiographical information
- diary, journal, log of daily events
- calendar
- daily schedule
- things-to-do list
- transportation information
- medication information and checklist
- photographs and names of therapists, physicians
- timeline of recent relevant medical history

The outside of the notebook should be clearly labeled for easy identification, and a pencil and/or pen should be attached to the inside front cover. Sohlberg and Mateer (1989b) describe a structured training program for teaching use of the notebook, starting with basic identification of sections of the book and leading up to initiation of independent use of the book for a variety of purposes.

Everyday materials such as colored key jackets and "sticky" notes should not be overlooked as valuable external memory aids; individual therapists can incorporate these to remedy specific problems identified with the patient and can also refer to Harrell et al. (1992) and Parenté and Herrmann (1996) for additional creative uses of these and other common items.

External aid devices particularly relevant for patients with communication and memory impairments include electronic devices for finding words and checking spelling and any devices for storage of other verbal material difficult to retrieve due to lack of contextual associations (e.g., names, phone numbers, medication names and doses). For patients with difficulty reading, recalling, or correctly dialing telephone numbers, portable devices can "look up" the number and provide electronic tones to bypass the necessity for dialing.

Prospective memory aids include alarm watches, timers, and other (usually electronic) devices for providing reminders to perform activities at specific times. Some "voice memo" devices record brief messages and can also be programmed to signal the patient to play back the recordings at specific times, thus addressing both the time-specific and content-specific aspects of prospective memory demands. Parenté and Herrmann (1996) describe other types of reminder devices or systems, including the Appointment Minder, which beeps to remind the patient to check the appointment book, and the Neuropage system (Hersh & Treadgold, 1994), which utilizes a computer programmed to notify the patient, by pager, of upcoming appointments.

While the temptation is strong to encourage patients to make full use of capabilities of elaborate electronic devices, the therapist is cautioned to carefully assess the patient's current level of functioning as well as specific memory needs in designing appropriate training in aids use. Most electronic data storage devices and alarm watches first require programming by the therapist or caregiver for specific purposes, for patients with significant memory impairments, followed by patients then being taught to independently use the devices and the stored information.

•   •   •

Memory disturbance ranks high among persistent deficits in patients with brain injury. Impairments in LTM processes are manifested in deficits of encoding, consolidation, and retrieval of new information, as well as in retrieval of stored remote memories relevant to functional behavior. The nature of the specific neurological results in cases of traumatic brain injury (multiple lesions, subcortical damage, frequent temporal and frontal lobe involvement) contributes to the complexity of the cognitive deficits seen in such cases.

Treatment planning should address the sources of presenting problems, the nature of presenting functional limitations, and the patient's and caregiver's needs in rehabilitation outcome. Finally, therapeutic approaches must be realistic and based on research findings. Traditional and still-popular restorative approaches to memory and communication rehabilitation produce limited, if any, improvement in process-level impairments and have minimal effect on functional-level deficits. The most effective rehabilitative treatment program relies on combinations of training in personal compensatory strategies, training in the use of external aids, and domain-specific training.

REFERENCES

Acker, M.B. (1990). A review of the ecological validity of neuropsychological tests. In D.E. Tupper & K.D. Cicerone (Eds.), *The neuropsychology of everyday life: Assessment and basic competencies* (pp. 19–55). Boston: Kluwer.

Adams, J., Graham, D., & Gennarelli, T. (1985). Contemporary neuropathological considerations regarding brain damage in head injury. In D. Becker & J. Povlishack (Eds.), *Central nervous system trauma status report: 1985*. Washington, DC: National Institutes of Health, National Institute for Neurological and Communicative Disorders and Stroke.

Baddeley, A., & Hitch, G. (1974). Working memory. In G. Bower (Ed.), *Recent advances in learning and motivation*. New York: Academic Press.

Bigler, E. (1990). Neuropathology of traumatic brain injury. In E. Bigler (Ed.), *Traumatic brain injury*. Austin, TX: PRO-ED.

Bracy, O.L. (1986). Cognitive rehabilitation: A process approach. *Cognitive Rehabilitation, 4*, 10–17.

Broadbent, D.E., Cooper, P.F., Fitzgerald, P., & Parkes, K.R. (1982). The cognitive failures questionnaire (CFQ) and its correlates. *British Journal of Clinical Psychology, 21*, 1–16.

Brooks, N. (1984). Cognitive deficits after head injury. In N. Brooks (Ed.), *Closed head injury*. Oxford, England: Oxford University Press.

Cowan, N. (1996). Short-term memory, working memory, and their importance in language processing. *Topics in Language Disorders 17*, 1–18.

Crosson, B., Barco, P., Velozo, C., Bolesta, M., Werts, D., & Brobeck, T. (1989). Awareness and compensation in post-acute head injury rehabilitation. *Journal of Head Trauma Rehabilitation, 4*, 46–54.

Ehrlich, J., & Sipes, A. (1985). Group treatment of communication skills for head trauma patients. *Cognitive Rehabilitation*, 32–37.

Gabrieli, J., McGlinchey-Berroth, R., Carrillo, M., Cermak, L., & Disterhoft, J. (1995). Intact delay-eyeblink classical conditioning in amnesia. *Behavioral Neurosciences, 109*, 819–827.

Glisky, E., & Schacter, D. (1987). Acquisition of domain specific knowledge in organic amnesia: Training for computer related work. *Neuropsychologia, 25*, 893–906.

Harrell, M., Parenté, F., Bellingrath, E., & Lisicia, K. (1992). *Cognitive rehabilitation of memory: A practical guide*. Gaithersburg, MD: Aspen Publishers, Inc.

Hartley, L. (1995). *Cognitive-communication abilities following brain injury*. San Diego, CA: Singular Publishing.

Hersh, N., & Treadgold, L. (1994). Neuropage: The rehabilitation of memory dysfunction by prosthetic memory aid cuing. *Neurorehabilitation, 4*, 187–197.

Hutchinson, J. (1993). *Components of cognitive rehabilitation*. Presented at the Society for Cognitive Rehabilitation, First Annual Training Seminar, Atlanta, GA.

Hutchinson, J., & Watkins, M. (1994). *TRACES: An adjustable memory strategy*. Presented at the Cognitive Rehabilitation and Community Integration Conference, San Antonio, TX.

Knowlton, B., Mangels, J., & Squire, L. (1996). A neostriatal learning system in humans. *Science, 273*, 1399–1402.

Lawton, M.P., & Brody, E.M. (1969). Assessment of older people: Self-maintaining and instrumental activities of daily living. *Gerontologist, 9*, 179–186.

Lezak, M. (1995). *Neuropsychological assessment*. New York: Oxford.

Markowitsch, H. (1995). Which brain regions are critically involved in the retrieval of old episodic memory? *Brain Research Reviews, 21*, 117–127.

Mateer, C.A., Sohlberg, M.M., & Crineon, J. (1987). Perceptions of memory function in individuals with closed-head injury. *Journal of Head Trauma Rehabilitation, 2*, 74–84.

Mattiolli, F., Grassi, F., Perani, D., Cappa, S., Miozzo, A., & Fazio, F. (1996). Persistent post-traumatic retrograde amnesia: A neuropsychological and (18)FDG PET study. *Cortex, 32*, 121–129.

McKinlay, W., Brooks, D., Martinage, E., & Marshall, M. (1981). The short-term outcome of severe blunt head injury as reported by relatives of the injured persons. *Journal of Neurology, Neurosurgery and Psychiatry, 44*, 527.

Parenté, R., & Anderson-Parenté, J. (1991). *Retraining memory: Techniques and applications*. Houston, TX: CSY.

Parenté, R., & Herrmann, D. (1996). *Retraining cognition: Techniques and applications*. Gaithersburg, MD: Aspen Publishers, Inc.

Parenté, R., Twum, M., & Zoltan, B. (1994). Transfer and generalization of cognitive skills after traumatic brain injury. *Neurorehabilitation, 4*, 25–35.

Prigatano, G. (1990). Effective traumatic brain injury rehabilitation: Team/patient interaction. In E. Bigler (Ed.), *Traumatic brain injury* (pp. 297–312). Austin, TX: PRO-ED.

Prigatano, G.P., Fordyce, D.J., Zeiner, H.K., Roueche, J.R., Pepping, M., & Wood, B.C. (1984). Neuropsychological rehabilitation after closed head injury in young adults. *Journal of Neurology, Neurosurgery and Psychiatry, 47*, 505–513.

Reisberg, B., & Ferris, S.H. (1982). Diagnosis and assessment of the older patient. *Hospital and Community Psychiatry, 33*, 104–110.

Rempel-Clower, N., Zola, S., Squire, L., & Amaral, D. (1996). Three cases of enduring memory impairment after bilateral damage limited to the hippocampal formation. *Journal of Neuroscience, 16*, 5233–5255.

Richardson, J. (1995). The efficacy of imagery mnemonics in memory remediation. *Neuropsychologia, 33*, 1345–1357.

Sohlberg, M., & Mateer, C. (1987). Effectiveness of an attention training program. *Journal of Clinical and Experimental Neuropsychology, 9*, 117–130.

Sohlberg, M., & Mateer, C. (1989a). The assessment of cognitive-communicative functions in head injury. *Topics in Language Disorders, 9*, 15–33.

Sohlberg, M., & Mateer, C. (1989b). *Introduction to cognitive rehabilitation: Theory and practice*. New York: Guilford Press.

Squire, L., & Alvarez, P. (1995). Retrograde amnesia and memory consolidation: A neurobiological perspective. *Current Opinions in Neurobiology, 5*, 169–177.

Sunderland, A., Harris, J.E., & Gleave, J. (1984). Memory failures in everyday life following severe head injury. *Journal of Clinical and Experimental Neuropsychology, 6*, 127–142.

Tuokko, H., & Crockett, D. (1991). Assessment of everyday functioning in normal and malignant memory disordered elderly. In D. Tupper & K. Cicerone (Eds.), *The neuropsychology of everyday life*. Boston: Kluwer.

Uzzell, B.P., Obrist, W.D., Dolinskas, C.A., & Langfitt, T.W. (1986). Relationship of acute CBF and ICP findings to neuropsychological outcome in head injury. *Journal of Neurosurgery, 65*, 630–635.

Wilson, B. (1987). *Rehabilitation of memory*. New York: Guilford Press.

Wilson, B., Cockburn, J., Baddeley, A., & Hiorns, R. (1989). Development and validation of a test battery for detecting and monitoring everyday memory problems. *Journal of Experimental Neuropsychology, 11*, 855–870.

Ylvisaker, M., & Holland, A. (1985). Coaching, self-coaching, and rehabilitation of head injury. In D. Johns (Ed.), *Clinical management of neurogenic communicative disorders* (2nd ed.). Boston: Little, Brown.

Zasler, N.D. (1991). Pharmacological aspects of cognitive function following traumatic brain injury. In J.S. Kreutzer & P. Wehman (Eds.), *Cognitive rehabilitation for persons with traumatic brain injury: A functional approach* (pp. 87–94). Baltimore: Paul H. Brookes Publishing.

11

Memory Impairments Underlying Language Difficulties in Dementia

Tamiko Azuma and Kathryn A. Bayles

The essential and often earliest feature of dementia is memory impairment. The *Diagnostic and Statistical Manual of Mental Disorders*, 4th edition (DSM-IV; American Psychiatric Association, 1994), used by many clinicians to make the diagnosis of dementia, lists memory disorder as a primary characteristic of dementia. Along with impaired memory, individuals also must display at least one of the following: aphasia, apraxia, agnosia, or disturbance in executive function.

Perhaps the most devastating consequence of dementia, to both caregivers and patients, is the progressive decline in communicative ability resulting from deteriorating memory and intellect. Alzheimer's disease (AD) is the most common cause of dementia, although it is associated with many other diseases, among them vascular disease, Parkinson's disease (PD), Huntington's disease, Pick's disease, and Lewy body disease (LBD).

This work was supported, in part, by National Multipurpose Research and Training Center Grant 5 P60 DC-01409-05 from the National Institute on Deafness and Other Communication Disorders, National Institutes of Health. We gratefully acknowledge Cheryl Tomoeda, Jody Wood, and Robyn Cruz. Correspondence regarding this chapter should be addressed to either the first author at: Department of Psychology, Box 871104, Arizona State University, Tempe, AZ 85287-1104 (e-mail: azuma@cnet.shs.arizona.edu), or the second author at: Institute for Neurogenic Communication Disorders, Department of Speech and Hearing Sciences, PO Box 210071, The University of Arizona, Tucson, AZ 85721-0071.

Top Lang Disord 1997;18(1):58–71

Almost all patients with dementia display some type of language dysfunction, such as difficulty in following and participating in conversations. Most of the linguistic communication deficits of dementia patients are reducible to underlying memory impairments.

This chapter describes the memory profiles of patients with different dementia-producing diseases, the impact of memory deficits on language, some of the individual tests and test batteries used to assess memory and language impairments, and several strategies for facilitating language in dementia patients. It would be impossible to review the language and memory problems of all types of dementia-associated diseases in one brief chapter; thus, the scope of this chapter is limited to a discussion of AD, the most common of the cortical dementias; PD, the most common of the subcortical dementias; and LBD, which typically results in both cortical and subcortical neuropathology. Understanding the patterns of impaired and preserved memory functions in dementia patients and their impact on communicative ability can lead to the development of more effective assessment techniques and clinical interventions.

GENERAL MEMORY PROFILES OF INDIVIDUALS WITH AD, PD, AND LBD

Alzheimer's disease

In the earliest stages and throughout its course, AD is characterized by impaired memory of specific events, also known as *episodic memory* (e.g., Bayles, 1991; Bayles & Kaszniak, 1987; Folstein & Powell, 1984). Episodic memory is considered a subsystem of *declarative memory*, the memory system that includes consciously learned, fact-based knowledge (Tulving, 1972, 1983). Episodic memory consists of information about temporally dated episodes in a person's life. The most commonly reported first symptom of AD is complaint of memory problems (Bayles, 1991). Individuals in the early stages of the disease will forget recent personal events, such as the previous night's activities or the location of their car in a parking lot. With increasing severity, patients show deficits in other declarative memory systems, namely semantic and lexical memory (Bayles & Kaszniak, 1987; Becker & Lopez, 1992). *Semantic memory* refers to knowledge about concepts, and *lexical memory* is knowledge about words. Clearly, these bodies of knowledge are interrelated, but they are separable.

Consider that people can think of concepts for which they have no words. In contrast to declarative memory deficits, skills that are dependent on procedural memory remain intact. *Procedural memory* includes knowledge of the process or procedures of various actions. This knowledge can be so well learned that the procedures are performed automatically, such as in typing or tying a shoe. Another memory system affected in AD patients is *working memory*, the system responsible for activating and retrieving relevant knowledge and focusing attention (Baddeley, 1986).

The neuropathology of AD, which includes the presence of neurofibrillary tangles, neuritic plaques, and areas of granulovacuolar degeneration, affects brain areas that are important for memory (Bayles, 1993; Bayles & Kaszniak, 1987; Becker & Lopez, 1992). It is believed that the deficits in episodic memory reflect neuropathological changes in the hippocampal complex, and deficits in semantic memory result from disease in cortical association areas. Procedural memory, on the other hand, is believed to remain intact because the basal ganglia and associated structures are relatively free of disease (Bayles, 1993).

Parkinson's disease

Dementia can occur in PD, but it is somewhat infrequent. It is important to note that AD pathology is more frequently observed in PD patients than in the general population. Thus, some PD patients with dementia are likely to have AD neuropathology. Current estimates of dementia rates in PD range between 10% and 20% (Girotti et al., 1988; Lees, 1985; Mayeux et al., 1988; Tison et al., 1995). The general memory and language profile of PD patients with dementia is similar to that of AD patients, except the decline in communicative function is more gradual (Gainotti, Caltagirone, Massullo, & Miceli, 1980; Levin & Tomer, 1992; Mahurin, Feher, Nance, Levy, & Pirozzolo, 1993). Recent research indicates that the cognitive decline of PD patients is relatively slow (Bayles et al., 1996). Similar to AD patients, PD patients with dementia show deficits in episodic, semantic, and lexical memory. However, PD also is commonly associated with impaired procedural memory, even in those individuals without dementia (Saint-Cyr, Taylor, & Lang, 1988; Taylor & Saint-Cyr, 1995). The procedural memory deficits are thought to result from disease effects in the basal ganglia (Bayles, 1993; Saint-Cyr et al., 1988). Thus, PD dementia patients show deficits in both procedural and declarative memory systems.

Lewy body disease

LBD was previously thought to be a relatively rare form of dementia, but some researchers now propose that it is one of the more common forms (Burns, Luthert, Levy, Jacoby, & Lantos, 1990; Homer et al., 1988). Patients with LBD often have concomitant AD pathology, and it has been proposed that LBD is a variant of AD. However, there are reported cases of patients with "pure" LBD without the characteristic neuropathology of AD, and some researchers argue that LBD is neuropathologically distinct from AD (see Cercy & Bylsma, 1997, for a review). This disease is characterized by the presence of Lewy bodies, protein deposits with a granular central core surrounded by a halo, in cortical regions.

As with AD patients, the earliest and most prominent feature of LBD is episodic memory impairment, and, with increasing severity, cognitive deficits become widespread. Although there are few formal neuropsychological studies of LBD patients, their cognitive profile has been reported to be comparable to AD patients, and LBD patients often are initially diagnosed with probable AD (Hansen et al., 1990). In the early stages, LBD patients generally suffer less cognitive impairment than early AD patients (Maxim & Bryan, 1996; Salmon et al., 1996). The observed deficits in episodic, semantic, and lexical memory and other cognitive functions are proposed to reflect neuropathological abnormalities in the neocortex of the temporal, frontal, and parietal lobes (Salmon et al., 1996).

The neuropathologies associated with these diseases are obviously complex. However, their impact on cognition is similar in that most patients with these diseases have memory and language deficits severe enough to warrant a diagnosis of dementia.

THE IMPACT OF DEMENTIA ON LANGUAGE ABILITIES

As previously mentioned, dementia patients experience progressive deficits in working memory and semantic, episodic, and lexical subsystems of declarative memory. These memory impairments are reflected in the language of such patients. Individuals with dementia show poor auditory comprehension, poor topic maintenance, reference errors, sentence fragments in their spoken discourse, and difficulty formulating and remembering the content of sentences (Appell, Kertesz, & Fisman, 1982; Bayles & Kaszniak, 1987;

Kempler, Curtiss, & Jackson, 1987; Schwartz, Marin, & Saffran, 1979; Tomoeda, Bayles, Trosset, Azuma, & McGeagh, 1996).

However, the grammar and pronunciation of patients' spoken discourse remain good, indicating that syntactic and phonological knowledge is intact. Indeed, the syntactic complexity of their sentences is comparable to that of unimpaired individuals (Appell et al., 1982; Hier, Hagenlocker, & Shindler, 1985; Kempler et al., 1987; Schwartz et al., 1979). Dementia patients also can recognize and spontaneously correct syntactic errors (Whitaker, 1976). For example, if they are told the sentence, "He called he mother," they can recognize that the sentence is incorrect and say the sentence correctly ("He called his mother"). They maintain the ability to read aloud, even in the advanced stages of the disease, when the ability to understand written material is lost (Bayles, Tomoeda, & Trosset, 1993; Hart, Smith, & Swash, 1986).

Although the language of dementia patients indicates that the *form* of language, such as knowledge of syntax and phonology, remains intact, there are deficits in *semantics*, the meaning aspects of language. Individuals with dementia are deficient in the use and comprehension of the meaning, reference, and pragmatic (contextual) aspects of language. The spoken and written discourse of mild dementia patients is impoverished in meaningful content (Tomoeda et al., 1996). With moderate and severe dementia, the discourse increasingly contains empty phrases and bizarre content (Appell et al., 1982; Bayles, Tomoeda, Kaszniak, Stern, & Eagans, 1985; Hier et al., 1985; Nicholas, Obler, Albert, & Helm-Estabrooks, 1985). Dementia patients also experience increasing difficulty in naming objects and defining concepts.

The Global Deterioration Scale (GDS; Reisberg, Ferris, de Leon, & Crook, 1982) was developed to profile the cognitive/functional abilities of patients in different stages of dementia severity. The degree of linguistic impairment experienced by dementia patients varies with the degree of dementia severity as demonstrated by the following GDS descriptions of communicative function. In the early confusional stage, Stage 3, the impact of memory deficits on communicative ability are relatively subtle. Affected individuals often will forget what they were about to say and experience some word-finding (word-retrieval) problems, but the form of their language remains intact (i.e., syntax and phonology are correct). In Stage 4, the late confusional stage, individuals have good reading and auditory comprehension but rapidly forget the information. They still have intact language form but continue to have problems with word retrieval. When individuals are classified as GDS Stage 5, or early dementia, language difficulties are more pronounced. Patients produce less spontaneous language, and spoken discourse reveals a limited vocabulary with less cohesion between sentences. However, they can still answer yes/no and multiple-choice questions and can carry on simple conversations. In Stage 6, patients demonstrate obvious language and memory difficulties. The content of their language is severely affected, although the form of their language remains intact. Their spontaneous language is limited and contains many empty and/or bizarre phrases. The auditory and written comprehension of these individuals is poor. In GDS Stage 7, patients are characterized by global cognitive deficits. At this stage, the form of language is impaired and their spontaneous language contains almost no meaningful content. By Stage 8, individuals show little or no oral or written abilities.

These descriptions by the authors of the GDS show that many language deficits exhibited by dementia patients arise from underlying memory impairments. However, it also is clear that the impact of dementia on communicative abilities can vary widely, ranging from relatively subtle word-finding difficulties in the early stages to profoundly impaired (or absent) language in the later stages. An important issue is how to assess the impairments of language and memory in dementia patients across this range of severity.

TECHNIQUES FOR ASSESSING LANGUAGE AND MEMORY IMPAIRMENTS IN DEMENTIA

Several tests are used to assess the impact of dementia on cognitive abilities, particularly on language and memory. These tests range from short, individual tests to test batteries, which contain several subtests and are standardized for individuals with and without dementia. In the next section, some of the more commonly used individual tests and test batteries are reviewed.

Individual tests

Individual tests are frequently used to assess language abilities of dementia patients because they are sensitive to dementia severity, they are short, and they are easily administered. Among the most commonly used tasks are the *confrontation naming* and *verbal fluency* (a.k.a. *generative naming*) tasks.

Probably the most widely used confrontation naming test is the Boston Naming Test (BNT; Kaplan, Goodglass, & Weintraub, 1983). In this task, individuals are asked to name black-and-white line drawings of objects. The version of the BNT usually administered to dementia patients includes 60 items, although a shorter, 15-item version also is reported to be sensitive to dementia (Morris et al., 1989). The BNT items range in word frequency and, thus, vary in difficulty. A recently developed naming test, the Armstrong Naming Test (Armstrong, 1996), also contains items that range in familiarity and has successfully distinguished AD patients from unimpaired older adults.

Object misnaming is commonly observed in dementia patients (e.g., Appell et al., 1982; Bayles & Boone, 1982; Bayles & Tomoeda, 1983; Flicker, Ferris, Crook, & Bartus, 1987; Kirshner, Webb, Kelly, & Wells, 1984; Martin & Fedio, 1983; Schwartz et al., 1979). Although no-dementia PD patients are not impaired in naming, PD patients with dementia are reported to have mild naming impairments (Cummings, Darkins, Mendez, Hill, & Benson, 1988; Fisher, Gatterer, & Danielczyk, 1988; Globus, Mildworf, & Melamed, 1985; Matison, Mayeux, Rosen, & Fahn, 1982). LBD patients also display a mild confrontation naming deficit (Salmon et al., 1996). In general, confrontation naming ability diminishes as dementia severity increases (Martin & Fedio, 1983).

Another popular test of language and memory is the verbal fluency task. Two types of verbal fluency tasks are used: (1) semantic and (2) letter verbal fluency. In semantic verbal fluency tasks, individuals are given one minute to produce items from a given category. A typical category would be "animals," and responses may include "dog, cat, cow, lamb, deer, [etc]." In letter verbal fluency tasks, individuals are given one minute to provide words that begin with a particular letter. For example, given the letter *S,* an individual may provide, "slide, sad, silly, sing, sword, [etc.]." The Controlled Oral Word Association Test (a.k.a. the FAS test; Borkowski, Benton, & Spreen, 1967) from the Multilingual Aphasia Examination (Benton & Hamsher, 1983) is a commonly used letter fluency task. In both tasks, performance is based on the number of correct responses provided by the patient.

These two verbal fluency tasks are very sensitive to dementia. It is commonly reported that PD and AD patients provide fewer responses than normal individuals (Appell et al., 1982; Bayles et al., 1989; Bayles, Trosset, Tomoeda, Montgomery, & Wilson, 1993; Flicker et al., 1987; Flowers, Robertson, & Sheridan, 1996; Gurd & Ward, 1989; Martin & Fedio, 1983; Monsch et al., 1992; Randolph, Braun, Goldberg, & Chase, 1993; Raskin, Sliwinski, & Borod, 1992). Salmon and colleagues (1996) also report poor letter and semantic fluency performance for LBD patients.

Semantic fluency performance is usually thought to reflect the integrity of semantic memory because individuals must retrieve knowledge of concepts to complete the task. Therefore, the poor fluency performance of dementia patients, relative to unimpaired individuals, often is considered evidence of semantic memory impairment. It should be kept in mind, however, that verbal fluency tasks involve multiple memory systems. For example, impaired working memory could affect patients' ability to remember the current category or previously provided responses and cause deficient performance. Thus, this task may reflect deficits in semantic memory, lexical memory, working memory, and/or attention. Regardless of the specific processes involved, it is clear that verbal fluency tasks are extremely sensitive to cognitive impairments of dementia patients.

Test batteries

Although individual tests are convenient, they may not provide an adequate profile of a patient's memory and language functions. Test batteries are composed of multiple subtests and allow for a more fully developed composite of cognitive abilities. A difficulty in testing patients is that no single test battery can sufficiently assess language and memory across all stages of dementia because the range of impairments is so broad. A test sensitive to language deficits that discriminates mild dementia individuals from unimpaired individuals will be too difficult for more severe dementia patients. On the other hand, a test easy enough for severe dementia individuals will be too easy for mild dementia patients. If patients do not make any mistakes on the test, it is not sensitive to their impaired functions. Recently, two measures have been developed expressly for measuring the communicative abilities of dementia patients: the Arizona Battery for Communicative Disorders of Dementia (ABCD; Bayles & Tomoeda, 1993) and the Functional Linguistic Communication Inventory (FLCI; Bayles & Tomoeda, 1994).

Arizona Battery for Communicative Disorders of Dementia

This test battery was designed to assess language and related cognitive abilities of mild to moderate dementia patients. This battery includes 17 subtests that evaluate five general areas: (1) episodic memory, (2) linguistic expression, (3) linguistic comprehension, (4) mental status, and (5) visuospatial construction. Fourteen of the tests were specifically designed to measure memory and language skills. Episodic memory is assessed using a story-retelling task with both immediate and delayed retelling, and a word learning task, which tests the free recall, cued recall, and recognition of words. Linguistic expression is evaluated by performance on object description (of a nail), verbal fluency, confrontation naming, and concept definition tests. The tests of linguistic comprehension include following commands, comparative questions, repetition, and reading comprehension of words and sentences.

The ABCD overall performance score is highly effective for screening mild and moderate AD patients from unimpaired older adults (Bayles & Tomoeda, 1993), and its discrimination is superior to performance on several individual tests, including the Mini-Mental State Examination (Folstein, Folstein, & McHugh, 1975) and verbal fluency tests. The validity and reliability of the ABCD has been established and standardized for both AD and PD patients.

In addition to the overall performance score, some of the subtest performances have proven to be especially sensitive to dementia, particularly the episodic memory tests: story retelling with immediate and delayed retelling, and word learning total recall. In the story-retelling test, patients are told a short story. Immediately afterward, they are asked to tell the story back to the examiner (immediate retelling), then, after a short distractor task, they again are asked to tell the story (delayed retelling). The entire test takes only about five minutes to administer. The story-retelling performance scores correctly classified 83% of mild AD patients, 100% of moderate AD patients, and 92% of older adults without AD (Bayles & Tomoeda, 1993). The word learning test involves multiple stages. In the first word learning stage, patients are asked category questions about visually presented words (presented in blocks of four). In the free-recall stage, the patients recall as many words as they can from the word learning stage. In the cued-recall stage, the examiner provides category cues for any words not previously recalled. The combined performance in the free- and cued-recall stages (i.e., the total recall score) correctly classified 93% of mild AD patients, 98% of moderate AD patients, and 93% of older adults without AD.

It is logical that these episodic memory tests are particularly sensitive to dementia because episodic memory is impaired early and throughout the progression of dementia. One limitation of the ABCD is that it is not appropriate for patients with severe dementia because of floor effects in their performance, particularly on the verbal episodic memory tests. In other words, the severe dementia patients are unable to perform the tasks at all, so it is not possible to draw meaningful conclusions from their performance.

Functional Linguistic Communication Inventory

The FLCI (Bayles & Tomoeda, 1994) was designed to assess the functional communicative abilities of patients with more severe dementia. The subtests of the FLCI measure patients' ability to greet and name, answer questions, write, comprehend signs, match objects to pictures, read and comprehend single words, reminisce, follow commands, pantomime, gesture, and carry on conversations. There are no explicit tests of episodic memory because the memory deficits of severe dementia individuals are so profound that they often cannot perform such tests. Although the semantic and lexical memory systems also are impaired, patients can still perform many simple language tests. This test battery is sensitive to differences in patients with moderate, moderately severe, severe, and very severe dementia (Bayles & Tomoeda, 1994). With its established validity and reliability, the FLCI is useful for testing the preserved functional communicative abilities of individuals with more severe dementia.

Recent test batteries

Two of the newest test batteries developed to assess the language/memory abilities of individuals with neurological disorders are the Multidisciplinary Cognitive Assessment System (MCAS; Idelkope, Hollenbeck, & Spencer, 1997) and the Scales of Adult Independence, Language, and Recall (SAILR; Sonies, 1997). The MCAS contains a set of tests designed to assess cognitive-linguistic abilities and includes tests of verbal and written memory, reading, writing, and comprehension. The SAILR was developed to assess the functional independence of patients using separate interviews with the patient and the caregiver. This test battery also has subtests for evaluating patients' cognitive-linguistic abilities, particularly memory. These subtests include comprehension and recall of both sentences and paragraphs and expressive naming of pictures.

The previously described tests are among the most commonly used techniques for assessing the language and memory of dementia patients. The individual tests that are most sensitive to the memory deficits in dementia patients are summarized in Table 1.

Table 1. Summary of tests for assessing memory of dementia patients

Memory/ language measures	Examples of specific tests	Procedure	Memory systems evaluated
Confrontation naming	Boston Naming Test	Patient names line drawings of objects.	Semantic memory Lexical memory
Semantic verbal fluency	Animals, fruits	Patient produces items from a semantic category.	Semantic memory Working memory
Letter verbal fluency	FAS test of verbal fluency	Patient produces words starting with a particular letter.	Lexical memory Working memory
Immediate story retelling	Story-Retelling Immediate subtest of the ABCD Story-Retelling	Patient is told a short story and then asked to retell the story.	Episodic memory
Delayed story retelling	Delayed subtest of the ABCD	Patient is asked to retell a previously heard story after a brief delay.	Episodic memory
Recall of words	Word Learning Total Recall subtest of the ABCD	Patient is asked questions about a list of words and, later, recalls the words.	Episodic memory

STRATEGIES FOR FACILITATING LANGUAGE IN DEMENTIA PATIENTS

After assessment of the language and memory impairments of dementia patients, the next step is to develop strategies that can improve their language comprehension and production. The goal for clinicians is to create situations in which patients can access various memory systems with less effort. This can be accomplished by reducing demands on the impaired working and declarative memory systems (episodic and semantic memory), and increasing reliance on intact procedural and recognition memory. Although the strategies discussed in this section are most relevant to what is currently known about AD, in general, they are applicable to all forms of dementia.

To increase the conversational comprehension of dementia patients, one should use syntactically simple sentences because syntactically complex sentences are harder to process (Kemper, Anagnopoulos, Lyons, & Heberlein, 1994). For example, sentences with embedded clauses are more syntactically complex (e.g., "The woman who watched my dog last month is coming over tonight"). Also, shorter sentences phrased in the active form, rather than the passive, will reduce memory demands and be easier for patients to understand. As with unimpaired individuals, it is easier for dementia patients to comprehend high-frequency words than low-frequency words (Barker & Lawson, 1968; Kirshner et al., 1984; Wilson, Bacon, Kramer, Fox, & Kaszniak, 1983). Dementia patients also tend to use higher frequency words in their spontaneous speech, indicating that these words are more accessible. Whenever possible, one should use familiar words in place of low-frequency, unfamiliar words.

The familiarity of concepts can influence performance, and dementia patients have an easier time comprehending more familiar concepts. Patients are better at understanding, and are more likely to converse about, concepts or topics that are personally relevant or have been previously experienced (Snowden, Griffiths, & Neary, 1994). It is more difficult for them to discuss concepts they have only observed. For example, it will be easier for a dementia patient to talk or answer questions about a family member than about the leader of Russia. Patients also are more likely to actively participate in conversations that relate to events currently taking place or objects that are clearly visible. The episodic memory deficits associated with dementia cause a difficulty in recalling past events and in anticipating future events.

Certain forms (or wordings) of questions are easier for dementia patients to understand. Tasks or questions that require the active generation of information will be more difficult than those merely requiring recognition or selection among choices. Questions presented in a multiple-choice form (e.g., "Should we have spaghetti or chili for dinner?") or yes/no form ("Do you want spaghetti for dinner?") generally are easier. Open-ended, free-recall questions, such as "What movies have you seen recently?" require the patient to actively retrieve memories from episodic memory, an impaired system. As previously noted, dementia patients are deficient on verbal fluency tasks, tests that require the active retrieval of multiple items from semantic or lexical memory. Therefore, open-ended, generative questions, such as, "What should we have for dinner?" will be more difficult because patients must generate different possibilities and then compare (or search) those possibilities.

Dementia patients have trouble understanding discussions that require memory of previously stated propositions because their working memory is impaired. Therefore, long chains of reasoning or argument should be avoided. Instead, the speaker should present the gist of the argument in one or two sentences. With severe dementia patients, commands or procedures involving several steps should be broken down into single steps. This strategy decreases the load on working memory. Pronouns should be avoided because the listener must remember the referent of the pronoun across phrases and sentences. The memory demand is decreased if the speaker repeats the name or object in every statement.

Individuals with dementia have difficulty understanding statements in which contextual information (pragmatic knowledge) must be used for correct interpretations. Such statements are called *indirect statements/requests* because the intended meaning of the sentence is usually different from its literal meaning. For example, a dementia patient may not be able to interpret the statement, "I need some new clothes," into its intended meaning, "I want to go shopping." It is difficult to process these indirect statements because the listener must figure out the intent of the speaker. Indirect statements or requests should be replaced by statements that are direct and literal. When speaking with dementia patients, sarcasm, irony, and idiomatic expressions (especially slang) should be avoided because the intended meaning may not match the literal interpretation of the sentences.

Repetition of information also will facilitate comprehension. If sentences are repeated, it can help dementia patients overcome the impact of working memory deficits on spoken comprehension. Thus, dementia patients are more likely to remember and understand sentences if they are repeated throughout a conversation.

Most of these strategies were derived from the simple principle of reducing demands on impaired memory systems. Any technique that minimizes attentional and memory demands should facilitate the language abilities of individuals with dementia. These strategies for improving communicative function in dementia patients are listed in Table 2.

•   •   •

The impact of dementia on communicative abilities ranges from relatively subtle word-finding difficulties in the early stages to profoundly

Table 2. Strategies for facilitating language in dementia patients

Strategy	Avoid:	Use:
Use short sentences with simple syntax and in the active voice.	"The book read by John was good."	"John read a good book."
Use high-frequency words.	"The cinematography was simply superb!"	"The scenes in the movie were beautiful!"
Talk about experiences that are personal and familiar to the patient.	"What do you think about Boris Yeltsin?"	"Is your daughter well?"
Talk about current activities or visible objects rather than past or future events.	"What kind of crops did your father raise on his farm?"	"Do you like these flowers?" [Give flowers to patient.]
Avoid questions that require active recall. Use multiple choice or yes/no questions.	"What did you have last week for dinner?"	"Do you want spaghetti for dinner?"
Avoid pronouns.	"Bob told me that she's bringing it."	"Bob told me that Sara is bringing the dress."
With advanced dementia patients, break down commands into single steps.	"Write down your name on the green paper and hand it to me."	"Find the green paper. Now write your name. Please give it to me."
Avoid indirect requests/ statements. Be direct and literal.	"It seems like a nice day for shopping."	"Do you want to go shopping?"
Avoid sarcasm, ironic statements, and slang terms.	"He was really nice." [sarcastic tone]	"He was mean!"

impaired language in the later stages. Many language deficits observed in dementia patients are reducible to underlying memory impairments. Individuals with dementia display progressive impairments in semantic, episodic, and lexical memory. Dementia also results in working memory limitations. The most effective strategies for facilitating language comprehension and production in dementia patients are those that minimize attentional, working, and declarative memory demands.

REFERENCES

American Psychiatric Association (1994). *Diagnostic and statistical manual of mental disorders* (4th ed.). Washington, DC: Author.

Appell, J., Kertesz, A., & Fisman, M. (1982). A study of language functioning in Alzheimer's disease. *Brain and Language, 17*, 73–91.

Armstrong, L. (1996). Armstrong Naming Test. San Diego, CA: Singular Publishing.

Baddeley, A.D. (1986). *Working memory*. Oxford, England: Oxford University Press.

Barker, M.G., & Lawson, J.S. (1968). Nominal aphasia in dementia. *British Journal of Psychiatry, 114*, 1351–1356.

Bayles, K.A. (1991). Alzheimer's disease symptoms: Prevalence and order of appearance. *Journal of Applied Gerontology, 10*, 419–430.

Bayles, K.A. (1993). Pathology of language behavior in dementia. In G. Blanken, J. Dittman, H. Grimm, J. Marshall, & C. Wallesch (Eds.), *Linguistic disorders and pathologies: An international handbook*. New York: Walter de Gruyter.

Bayles, K.A., & Boone, D.R. (1982). The potential of language tasks for identifying senile dementia. *Journal of Speech and Hearing Research, 47*, 210–217.

Bayles, K.A., & Kaszniak, A.W. (1987). *Communication and cognition in normal aging and dementia*. Boston: Little, Brown.

Bayles, K.A., Salmon, D.P., Tomoeda, C.K., Jacobs, D., Caffrey, J.T., Kaszniak, A.W., & Troster, A.I. (1989). Semantic and letter category naming in Alzheimer's patients: A predictable difference. *Developmental Neuropsychology, 5*, 335–347.

Bayles, K.A., & Tomoeda, C.K. (1983). Confrontation naming impairment in dementia. *Brain and Language, 19*, 98–114.

Bayles, K.A., & Tomoeda, C.K. (1993). *The Arizona Battery for Communicative Disorders*. Tucson, AZ: Canyonlands Publishing.

Bayles, K.A., & Tomoeda, C.K. (1994). *The Functional Linguistic Communication Inventory*. Phoenix, AZ: Canyonlands Publishing.

Bayles, K.A., Tomoeda, C.K., Kaszniak, A.W., Stern, L.Z., & Eagans, K.K. (1985). Verbal perseveration of dementia patients. *Brain and Language, 25*, 102–116.

Bayles, K.A., Tomoeda, C.K., & Trosset, M.W. (1993). Alzheimer's disease: Effects on language. *Developmental Neuropsychology, 9*, 131–160.

Bayles, K.A., Tomoeda, C.K., Wood, J.A., Montgomery, E.B., Cruz, R.F., Azuma, T., & McGeagh, A. (1996). Change in cognitive function in idiopathic Parkinson's disease. *Archives of Neurology, 53*, 1140–1146.

Bayles, K.A., Trosset, M.W., Tomoeda, C.K., Montgomery, E.B., & Wilson, J. (1993). Generative naming in Parkinson's disease patients. *Journal of Clinical and Experimental Neuropsychology, 15*, 547–562.

Becker, J.T., & Lopez, O.L. (1992). Episodic memory in Alzheimer's disease: Breakdown of multiple memory processes. In L. Backman (Ed.), *Memory functioning in dementia* (pp. 27–43). Elsevier Science.

Benton, A., & Hamsher, K. (1983). *Multilingual Aphasia Examination.* Iowa City, IA: University of Iowa.

Borkowski, J.G., Benton, A.L., & Spreen, O. (1967). Word fluency and brain damage. *Neuropsychologia, 5,* 135–140.

Burns, A., Luthert, P., Levy, R., Jacoby, R., & Lantos, P. (1990). Accuracy of clinical diagnosis of Alzheimer's disease. *British Medical Journal, 301,* 1026.

Cercy, S.P., & Bylsma, F.W. (1997). Lewy bodies and progressive dementia: A critical review and meta-analysis. *Journal of the International Neuropsychological Society, 3,* 179–194.

Cummings, J.L., Darkins, A., Mendez, M., Hill, M.A., & Benson, D.F. (1988). Alzheimer's disease and Parkinson's disease: Comparison of speech and language alterations. *Neurology, 38,* 1556–1561.

Fisher, P., Gatterer, G., & Danielczyk, W. (1988). Semantic memory in DAT, MID, and parkinsonism. *Functional Neurology, 3,* 301–307.

Flicker, C., Ferris, S., Crook, T., & Bartus, R.T. (1987). Implications of memory and language dysfunction in naming deficits of senile dementia. *Brain and Language, 31,* 187–200.

Flowers, K.A., Robertson, C., & Sheridan, M.R. (1996). Some characteristics of word fluency in Parkinson's disease. *Journal of Neurolinguistics, 9,* 33–46.

Folstein, M.F., Folstein, S.E., & McHugh, P.R. (1975). "Mini-Mental State"; A practical method for grading the cognitive state of patients for the clinician. *Journal of Psychiatric Research, 12,* 189–198.

Folstein, M.F., & Powell, D. (1984). Is Alzheimer's disease inherited? A methodological review. *Integrated Psychiatry, 2,* 163–170.

Gainotti, G., Caltagirone, C., Massullo, C., & Miceli, G. (1980). Patterns of neuropsychologic impairment in various diagnostic groups of dementia. In L. Amaducci, A.N. Davison, & P. Antvono (Eds.), *Aging of brain and dementia* (pp. 245–250). New York: Raven Press.

Girotti, F., Solvieri, P., Carella, F., Piccolo, I., Caffarra, P., Musicco, M., & Caraceni, T. (1988). Dementia and cognitive impairment in Parkinson's disease. *Journal of Neurology, Neurosurgery and Psychiatry, 51,* 1498–1502.

Globus, M., Mildworf, B., & Melamed, E. (1985). Cerebral blood flow and cognitive impairment in Parkinson's disease. *Neurology, 35,* 1135–1139.

Gurd, J.M., & Ward, C.D. (1989). Retrieval from semantic and letter initial categories in patients with Parkinson's disease. *Neuropsychologia, 27,* 743–746.

Hansen, L., Salmon, D., Galasko, D., Masliah, E., Katzman, R., DeTeresa, R., Thal, L., Pay, M., Hofstetter, R., Klauber, M., Rice, V., Butters, N., & Alford, M. (1990). The Lewy body variant of AD: A clinical and pathologic entity. *Neurology, 40,* 1–8.

Hart, S., Smith, C.M., & Swash, M. (1986). Assessing intellectual deterioration. *British Journal of Clinical Psychology*, 25, 119–124.

Hier, D.B., Hagenlocker, K., & Shindler, A.G. (1985). Language disintegration in dementia: Effects of etiology and severity. *Brain and Language*, 25, 117–133.

Homer, A., Honovar, M., Lantos, P., Hastie, I., Kellett, J., & Millard, P. (1988). Diagnosing dementia: Do we get it right? *British Medical Journal*, 297, 894–896.

Idelkope, B., Hollenbeck, A., & Spencer, J. (1997). *Multidisciplinary Cognitive Assessment System (MCAS)*. Chicago: Applied Symbolix.

Kaplan, E., Goodglass, H., & Weintraub, S. (1983). *Boston Naming Test*. Philadelphia: Lea & Febiger.

Kemper, S., Anagnopoulos, C., Lyons, K., & Heberlein, W. (1994). Speech accommodations in dementia. *Journal of Gerontology: Psychological Sciences*, 49, 223–229.

Kempler, D., Curtiss, S., & Jackson, C. (1987). Syntactic preservation in Alzheimer's disease. *Journal of Speech and Hearing Research*, 30, 343–350.

Kirshner, H.S., Webb, W.G., Kelly, M.P., & Wells, C.E. (1984). Language disturbance: An initial symptom of cortical degeneration and dementia. *Archives of Neurology*, 41, 491–496.

Lees, A.J. (1985). Parkinson's disease and dementia. *Lancet*, 1, 43–44.

Levin, B.E., & Tomer, R. (1992). A prospective study of language abilities in Parkinson's disease. *Journal of Clinical and Experimental Neuropsychology*, 14, 34.

Mahurin, R.K., Feher, E.P., Nance, M.L., Levy, J.K., & Pirozzolo, F.J. (1993). Cognition in Parkinson's disease and related disorders. In R.W. Parks, R.F. Zec, & R.S. Wilson (Eds.), *Neuropsychology of Alzheimer's disease and other dementias* (pp. 308–349). New York: Oxford University Press.

Martin, A., & Fedio, P. (1983). Word production and comprehension in Alzheimer's disease: The breakdown of semantic knowledge. *Brain and Language*, 19, 124–141.

Matison, R., Mayeux, R., Rosen, J., & Fahn, S. (1982). "Tip-of-the-tongue" phenomenon in Parkinson's disease. *Neurology*, 32, 567–570.

Maxim, J., & Bryan, K. (1996). Language, cognition, and communication in older mentally ill people. In K. Bryan & J. Maxim (Eds.), *Communication disability and the psychiatry of old age*. San Diego, CA: Singular Publishing.

Mayeux, R., Stern, Y., Rosenstein, R., Marder, K., Hauser, A., Cote, L., & Fahn, S. (1988). An estimate of the prevalence of dementia in idiopathic Parkinson's disease. *Journal of Neurology, Neurosurgery and Psychiatry*, 45, 260–262.

Monsch, A.U., Bondi, M.W., Butters, N., Salmon, D.P., Katzman, R., & Thal, L.J. (1992). Comparisons of verbal fluency tasks in the detection of dementia of the Alzheimer's type. *Archives of Neurology*, 49, 1253–1258.

Morris, J.C., Heyman, A., Mohs, R.C., Hughes, J.P., van Belle, G., Fillenbaum, G., Mellits, E.D., Clark, C., & the CERAD Investigators. (1989). The consortium to establish a registry for Alzheimer's disease (CERAD): Part I. Clinical and neuropsychological assessment of Alzheimer's disease. *Neurology*, 39, 1159–1165.

Nicholas, M., Obler, L.K., Albert, M.S., & Helm-Estabrooks, N. (1985). Empty speech in Alzheimer's disease and fluent aphasia. *Journal of Speech and Hearing Research, 28,* 405–410.

Randolph, C., Braun, A.R., Goldberg, T.E., & Chase, T.N. (1993). Semantic fluency in Alzheimer's, Parkinson's, and Huntington's disease: Dissociation of storage and retrieval failures. *Neuropsychology, 7,* 82–88.

Raskin, S.A., Sliwinski, M., & Borod, J.C. (1992). Clustering strategies on tasks of verbal fluency in Parkinson's disease. *Neuropsychologia, 30,* 95–99.

Reisberg, B., Ferris, S.H., de Leon, M.J., & Crook, T. (1982). The Global Deterioration Scale (GDS): An instrument for the assessment of primary degenerative dementia (PDD). *American Journal of Psychiatry, 139,* 1136–1139.

Saint-Cyr, J.A., Taylor, A.E., & Lang, A.E. (1988). Procedural learning and neostriatal dysfunction in man. *Brain, 111,* 941–959.

Salmon, D.P., Galasko, D., Hansen, L.A., Masliah, E., Butters, N., Thal, L.F., & Katzman, R. (1996). Neuropsychological deficits associated with diffuse Lewy body disease. *Brain and Cognition, 31,* 148–165.

Schwartz, M.F., Marin, O.S.M., & Saffran, E.M. (1979). Dissociations of language function in dementia: A case study. *Brain and Language, 7,* 277–306.

Snowden, J., Griffiths, H., & Neary, D. (1994). Semantic dementia: Autobiographical contribution to preservation of meaning. *Cognitive Neuropsychology, 11,* 265–288.

Sonies, B. (1997). *Scales of Adult Independence, Language, and Recall.* Chicago: Riverside Publishing Company.

Taylor, A.E., & Saint-Cyr, J.A. (1995). The neuropsychology of Parkinson's disease. *Brain and Cognition, 28,* 281–296.

Tison, F., Dartigues, J.F., Auriacombe, S., Letenneur, L., Boller, F., & Alperovitch, A. (1995). Dementia in Parkinson's disease: A population based study in ambulatory and institutionalized individuals. *Neurology, 45,* 705–708.

Tomoeda, C.K., Bayles, K.A., Trosset, M.W., Azuma, T., & McGeagh, A. (1996). Cross sectional analysis of Alzheimer disease effects on oral discourse in a picture description task. *Alzheimer Disease and Associated Disorders, 10,* 204–215.

Tulving, E. (1972). Episodic and semantic memory. In E. Tulving & W. Donaldson (Eds.), *Organization of memory.* New York: Academic Press.

Tulving, E. (1983). *Elements of episodic memory.* Oxford, England: Oxford University Press.

Whitaker, H.A. (1976). A case of isolation of the language function. In H. Whitaker & H.A. Whitaker (Eds.), *Studies in neurolinguistics* (Vol. 2., pp. 1–58). New York: Academic Press.

Wilson, R.S., Bacon, L.D., Kramer, R.L., Fox, J.H., & Kaszniak, A.W. (1983). Word frequency effect and recognition memory in dementia of the Alzheimer type. *Journal of Clinical Neuropsychology, 5,* 97–104.

Putting Memory to Work in Language Intervention: Implications for Practitioners

Ronald B. Gillam

Researchers often disagree about the extent to which general cognitive mechanisms such as memory are involved in language acquisition. The authors that have contributed chapters to this book believe memory mechanisms play a critical role in normal language development and in situations, like language intervention, in which language is purposefully taught. This epilogue summarizes the role memory plays in language learning, describes a dynamic model of the relationships between working memory and long-term memory, and reviews intervention activities that promote memory and language development.

Consider some typical language intervention contexts:

- Connie, age 4, presents delayed expressive and receptive language development. Connie and her clinician play "restaurant" with toy people. As Connie pretends to feed a toy person, she says, "This boy eating." Her clinician offers a growth-relevant recast (Camarata, Nelson, & Camarata, 1994; Nelson, Camarata, Welsh, Butkovsky, & Camarata, 1996), saying, "Yes, that boy is eating."
- Tom, age 13, sustained a traumatic brain injury when he was involved in an automobile accident. He has recovered many of his language abilities but still has difficulties with narration. Tom and his clinician use a story schema diagram (Ylvisaker, 1995) as they write and revise stories.

Top Lang Disord 1997;18(1):72–79
© 1997 Aspen Publishers, Inc.

- John, age 64, is recovering from a left hemisphere stroke. John's clinician coaches him as he works through a script of a conversational interaction that involves ordering food at a restaurant (Holland & Beeson, 1995; Murray & Holland, 1995).

These three language intervention activities involve different language disorders, different aspects of language, and different levels of linguistic complexity. However, in each case, interactions between working memory and long-term memory processes are central to intervention efficacy. To be successful, these language learners must attend to what their clinicians say, construct mental representations of their clinicians' utterances, recall what they themselves usually say in the same context, detect a difference between the clinician's use of language and their use of language, realize that the difference is important, and then store this realization in a way that enables retrieval. Outside the therapy setting, learners need to activate their new-found language knowledge when they recognize similarities between the form–meaning–use interactions present in the current speaking context and the form–meaning–use interactions that were present in the therapy setting. From this perspective, it is clear that success in language intervention depends heavily on memory processes.

WORKING MEMORY AND LONG-TERM MEMORY

Figure 1 depicts a rather simple view of the dynamic relationships among working memory, long-term memory, information processing mechanisms, language ability, and world knowledge. Although this model does not represent all aspects of memory, it does include many of the mechanisms and relationships that are important for understanding the role that memory plays in language intervention.

There are four interrelated memory phases (encoding, storage, retrieval, and reporting) that occur simultaneously within long-term (relatively permanent) and working (ever-changing) memory. Learners represent information in their minds (encoding), hold it for immediate or later use (storage), access the information when they need it (retrieval), and communicate what they have remembered (reporting). The connections between these phases represent interdependencies among encoding, storage, retrieval, and reporting. For example, the way information is initially encoded affects the way it is stored, the kinds of cues that will be necessary

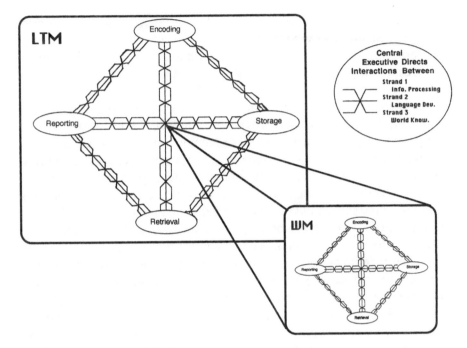

Figure 1. A basic model of memory.

for retrieval at a later time, and the amount of information that will be available for reporting (see Hudson & Gillam, Chapter 7, for a more complete discussion of dynamic relationships among memory phases during development).

The connections between the four memory phases are pictured as woven strands. One strand represents information processing abilities (e.g., attention, perception, and speed of processing), one represents language ability (phonological, lexical, syntactic, and discourse abilities), and one represents world knowledge or scripts (see Naremore, Chapter 8, for a discussion of scripts and their role in memory and language use). These processes work together to encode information, store it, retrieve it, and report it.

A central executive mechanism acts with respect to the learner's motivation and goals to influence interactions among these processes as they carry out the functions of the four memory phases. Learners who are driven to obtain a particular goal (e.g., more effective communication), who are more alert, who are faster processors, who have higher levels of language ability, and who have greater amounts of prior knowledge about a particular topic will encode, store, retrieve, and report information more completely and more efficiently than learners who are less motivated, who are less alert, who process information slowly, who have less complex language abilities, and/or who know less about the subject at hand.

Consistent with many other memory models (Cowan, 1995; Engle, Cantor, & Carullo, 1992; Ericsson & Kintsch, 1995; Just & Carpenter, 1992), working memory is depicted as those storage and processing functions within long-term memory that are active at a given moment. Working memory is not seen as a distinctly different kind of memory. Rather, it is the portion of long-term memory that is busy processing information. This processing involves simultaneously encoding information, storing it, retrieving related information that has already been stored, and reporting it.

Finally, the model assumes a general memory capacity that limits the amount of encoding, storage, retrieval, and reporting that can be accomplished at any given time. This general capacity is thought to result from the dynamic relationships among information processing functions, language abilities, and world knowledge. The capacity limitations that are often discussed in relationship to language impairment (Johnston, 1994; Montgomery, 1996, Chapter 2; Ellis Weismer, 1996, Chapter 3) are understood in this model to be the combined outcome of attention processes; speed of mental processing; phonological, lexical, syntactic, and discursive language knowledge; and general knowledge of the topic at hand. Some children may have deficiencies in one or two of these processes; others may have deficiencies in nearly all of these processes.

LANGUAGE AND MEMORY INTERVENTION

The earlier chapters on memory and language disorders have shown that language plays a critical role in memory and that memory plays a critical role in language. Therefore, it is difficult to separate language intervention from memory intervention. Activities done for the sake of improving language should have an impact on memory development just as activities done for the sake of improving memory should have an impact on language development.

Gillam and van Kleeck (1996, Chapter 5) suggest that intervention should primarily focus on social-interactive and academic uses of language in pragmatically relevant situations. However, within the larger context of functional intervention, learners can benefit from a temporary focus on particular aspects of language or cognition (Gillam, McFadden, & van Kleeck, 1995; Montgomery, 1996, Chapter 2). There are many intervention activities that benefit both memory and language. The following language intervention principles and activities are a sample of the clinical ideas that have been proposed in the earlier chapters.

1. Promote attention

Individuals with various kinds of language disorders evidence difficulties with attention (Campbell & McNeil, 1985; Loveland & Landry, 1986; Riddle, 1992; Tseng, McNeil, & Milenkovic, 1993). Following LaBerge (1995) and Cowan (1995), there are at least two attentional states that contribute to the client's encoding of the clinician's facilitative input. First, learners process information more quickly after they have preactivated relevant information in long-term memory. Second, encoding is enhanced when learners selectively attend to the most critical information.

Clinicians can mediate preparatory attention in older clients by communicating their intentions. For example, Tom's clinician might have started the session by reading the story they had composed during the previous session. Afterward, she could have increased Tom's preparatory attention by saying, "Today, we're going to expand on that story by adding information about the characters' plans for the actions they will take to solve their problems." When working with younger children, clinicians could influence preparatory attention by demonstrating the child's language targets three or four times within meaningful contexts. For example, Connie's clinician could have started the activity by asking her to watch and listen to him for a minute as he used the target structures while narrating his actions during play.

Clinicians can mediate selective attention by making the intervention targets as salient as possible and by limiting distractions. For example, Ellis Weismer, Hesketh, Hollar, and Neylon (1994) reported that children learned to produce novel words that clinicians had emphatically stressed better than novel words that had been produced with regular stress. These authors concluded that the emphatic stress helped direct the children's selective attention to new information to be learned. Increased selective attention appeared to influence children's encoding, recall, and reporting functions.

2. Speak clearly and slowly

Speech perception and speed of cognitive processing contribute to encoding. Some children with developmental language disorders have difficulties with perception of rapidly produced sounds (Sussman, 1993; Tallal, 1990; Tallal, Stark, & Mellitts, 1985) and with rapid cognitive processing (Johnston & Ellis Weismer, 1983; Sininger, Klatzky, & Kirchner, 1989). As noted by Ellis Weismer (Chapter 3), when clinicians slow their rates of speech, they provide learners with more time for processing, encoding, storage, and retrieval.

3. Promote phonological coding

Children with developmental language disorders frequently have difficulty with phonological aspects of encoding (Gillam, Cowan, & Day, 1995; Montgomery, 1995; Sussman, 1993). Montgomery (Chapter 2) and Fazio (Chapter 4) suggest teaching children nursery rhymes to help them develop phonological coding skills. Similarly, Gillam and van Kleeck (Chapter 5) found that children who received rhyming and phonological awareness training improved considerably on a measure of phonological coding ability.

Training in listening skills might also promote more efficient and elaborate encoding. Recently, Tallal and her colleagues (1996) have reported on a computer-assisted instruction program called Fast Forword that was designed to facilitate children's temporal processing abilities. At the present time, the authors' broad generalizations about the effectiveness of this intervention have yet to be empirically validated through careful experimentation and replication. Nonetheless, the efficacy data that have been reported (Tallal et al., 1996) appear promising. This intervention approach may be especially well-suited to facilitating selective attention to sound, maintenance of attention (or prolonged concentration), and phonological coding. If this proves to be the case, programs like Fast Forword should have an indirect impact on language development when they are instituted as a temporary focus on auditory processing within a larger program of functional language intervention.

4. Plan activities around topics or concepts that are familiar to the learner

Greater prior knowledge enables learners to attend more carefully to new information, which leads to more elaborate encoding, increased storage, and a greater variety of retrieval cues. Clinicians who wish to teach new language forms or new communicative functions should make optimal use of the learner's established scripts. This principle has been proposed for intervention with adults with dementia (Azuma & Bayles, Chapter 11), adolescents with language-based learning disabilities (Wynn-Dancy & Gillam, Chapter 9), and preschoolers with developmental language disorders (Naremore, Chapter 8).

5. Help learners organize new knowledge

Learners can remember much more information when they have organized their knowledge into meaningful chunks. For example, people struggle to recall 20 randomly presented letters, but they can easily remember 60 or 80 letters when the letters are part of words that compose sentences. Following the same logic, it makes sense to help learners organize new knowledge in ways that facilitate recall. Parenté and Herrmann (Chapter 6) suggest that clinicians teach categorization strategies to patients with head injury. Similarly, Hutchinson and Marquardt (Chapter 10) advise clinicians to practice specific recall strategies with their clients. Wynn-Dancy and Gillam (Chapter 9) describe learning strategies that help adolescents organize and recall information from readings and lectures. Montgomery (Chapter 2) suggests that practice with paraphrasing can help learners in the elementary grades use their own prior knowledge, vocabulary, and language structures that they are the most familiar with to organize new information.

6. Provide learners with retention cues

Clinicians need to build bridges between intervention targets and learners' knowledge and expectations. As suggested by Hudson and Gillam

(Chapter 7), clinician questions, summaries, drawings, and pictures can be internalized by learners as recall cues. Recall cues provided by clinicians, parents, or teachers can be very powerful. In some studies, children who were given retention cues during a novel experience had greater recall than children who did not receive extra cues as much as a year after the experience.

•   •   •

The primary point is that working memory, long-term memory, information processing mechanisms, language ability, and world knowledge are dynamically related in a system of learning. Language is essential in encoding, storage, retrieval, and reporting phases of memory, and memory is essential for language learning. As such, much of what is done in language intervention is, for all intents and purposes, also memory intervention. After many stimulating discussions with the authors who have contributed chapters to this volume, I am firmly convinced that clinicians should carefully consider relationships between language and memory as they devise individualized solutions to the language and learning problems encountered by the individuals they serve.

REFERENCES

Camarata, S.M., Nelson, K.E., & Camarata, M.N. (1994). Comparison of conversational-recasting and imitative procedures for training grammatical structures in children with specific language impairment. *Journal of Speech and Hearing Research, 37*(6), 1414–1423.

Campbell, T.F., & McNeil, M.R. (1985). Effects of presentation rate and divided attention on auditory comprehension in children with an acquired language disorder. *Journal of Speech and Hearing Research, 28*(4), 513–520.

Cowan, N. (1995). *Attention and memory: An integrated framework.* New York: Oxford University Press.

Ellis Weismer, S. (1996). Capacity limitations in working memory: The impact on lexical and morphological learning by children with language impairment. *Topics in Language Disorders, 17(1):* 33–44.

Ellis Weismer, S., Hesketh, L., Hollar, C., & Neylon, C. (1994). *The role of emphatic stress in lexical learning.* Poster presented at the annual convention of the American Speech-Hearing Association, New Orleans, LA.

Engle, R.W., Cantor, J., & Carullo, J.J. (1992). Individual differences in working memory and comprehension: A test of four hypotheses. *Journal of Experimental Psychology: Learning, Memory, and Cognition, 18*, 972–992.

Ericsson, K.A., & Kintsch, W. (1995). Long-term working memory. *Psychological Review, 102*(2), 211–245.

Fazio, B. (1996). Serial memory in children with specific language impairment: Examining specific content areas for assessment and intervention. *Topics in Language Disorders, 17*(1), 58–71.

Gillam, R.B., Cowan, N., & Day, L.S. (1995). Sequential memory in children with and without language impairment. *Journal of Speech and Hearing Research, 38,* 393–402.

Gillam, R.B., McFadden, T.U., & van Kleeck, A. (1995). Improving the narrative abilities of children with language disorders: Whole language and language skills approaches. In M. Fey, J. Windsor, & J. Reichle (Eds.), *Communication intervention for school-age children* (pp. 145–182). Baltimore: Paul H. Brookes Publishing.

Gillam, R.B., & van Kleeck, A. (1996). Phonological awareness training and short-term working memory: Clinical implications. *Topics in Language Disorders, 17*(1), 72–82.

Holland, A.L., & Beeson, P.M. (1995). Aphasia therapy. In H.S. Kirshner (Ed.), *Handbook of neurological speech and language disorders* (Vol. 33, pp. 445–463). New York: Marcel Dekker.

Johnston, J. (1994). Cognitive abilities of children with language impairment. In R.V. Watkins & M.L. Rice (Eds.), *Specific language impairments in children* (pp. 107–121). Baltimore: Paul H. Brookes Publishing.

Johnston, J.R., & Ellis Weismer, S. (1983). Mental rotation abilities in language-disordered children. *Journal of Speech and Hearing Research, 26,* 397–403.

Just, M.A., & Carpenter, P.A. (1992). A capacity theory of comprehension: Individual differences in working memory. *Psychological Review, 99,* 122–149.

LaBerge, D. (1995). *Attentional processing: The brain's art of mindfulness.* Cambridge, MA: Harvard University Press.

Loveland, K.A., & Landry, S.H. (1986). Joint attention and language in autism and developmental language delay. *Journal of Autism and Developmental Disorders, 16*(3), 335–349.

Montgomery, J. (1995). Examination of phonological working memory in specifically language impaired children. *Applied Psycholinguistics, 16,* 355–378.

Montgomery, J. (1996). Sentence comprehension and working memory in children with specific language impairment. *Topics in Language Disorders, 17*(1), 19–32.

Murray, L.L., & Holland, A.L. (1995). The language recovery of acutely aphasic patients receiving different therapy regimens. *Aphasiology, 9*(4), 397–405.

Nelson, K.E., Camarata, S.M., Welsh, J., Butkovsky, L., & Camarata, M. (1996). Effects of imitative and conversational recasting treatment on the acquisition of grammar in children with specific language impairment and younger language-normal children. *Journal of Speech and Hearing Research, 39*(4), 850–859.

Parenté, R., & Herrmann, D. (1996). Retraining memory strategies. *Topics in Language Disorders, 17*(1), 45–57.

Riddle, L.S. (1992). The attentional capacity of children with specific language impairment. *Dissertation Abstracts International, 53,* 6-B.

Sininger, Y.S., Klatzky, R.L., & Kirchner, D.M. (1989). Memory scanning speed in language-disordered children. *Journal of Speech and Hearing Research, 32*(2), 289–297.

Sussman, J.E. (1993). Perception of formant transition cues to place of articulation in children with language impairments. *Journal of Speech and Hearing Research, 36*(6), 1,286–1,299.

Tallal, P. (1990). Fine-grained discrimination deficits in language-learning impaired children are specific neither to the auditory modality nor to speech perception. *Journal of Speech and Hearing Research, 33*, 616–617.

Tallal, P., Miller, S.I., Bedi, G., Byma, G., Wang, X., Nagarajan, S.S., Schreiner, C., Jenkins, W.M., & Merzenich, M.M. (1996). Language comprehension in language-learning impaired children improved with acoustically modified speech. *Science, 271*, 81–84.

Tallal, P., Stark, R.E., & Mellitts, E.D. (1985). Identification of language-impaired children on the basis of rapid perception and production skills. *Brain and Language, 25*, 314–322.

Tseng, C.-H., McNeil, M.R., & Milenkovic, P. (1993). An investigation of attention allocation deficits in aphasia. *Brain and Language, 45*(2), 276–296.

Weismer, S.E. (1996). Capacity limitations on working memory: The impact on lexical and morphological learning by children with language impairment. *Topics in Language Disorders, 17*(1), 33–44.

Ylvisaker, M. (1995). Intervention for students with traumatic brain injury. In D.F. Tibbits (Ed.), *Language intervention: Beyond the primary grades* (pp. 313–372). Austin, TX: PRO-ED.

Index

M